Respiratory Medicine

Second Edition

D1306359

Respiratory Medicine

Second Edition

John J. Marini, M.D.
Associate Professor of Medicine
Vanderbilt University
Nashville, Tennessee

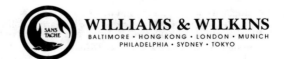

WILLIAMS & WILKINS
BALTIMORE · HONG KONG · LONDON · MUNICH
PHILADELPHIA · SYDNEY · TOKYO

Editor: Nancy Collins
Associate Editor: Carol Eckhart
Design: JoAnne Janowiak
Illustration Planning: Wayne Hubbel
Production: Raymond E. Reter

Copyright ©, 1987
Williams & Wilkins
428 East Preston Street
Baltimore, MD 21202, U.S.A.

Accurate indications, adverse reactions, and dosage schedules for drugs are provided in this book, but it is possible that they may change. The reader is urged to review the package information data of the manufacturers of the medications mentioned.

Printed in the United States of America
First Edition, 1981

Library of Congress Cataloging in Publication Data
Main entry under title:

Marini, John J.
   Respiratory medicine for the house officer.
   Rev. ed. of part of: Respiratory medicine and intensive care for the house officer. c1981.
   Includes bibliographies and index.
   1. Respiratory organs—Diseases.   I. Marini, John J. Respiratory medicine and intensive care for the house officer.   II. Title. [DNLM: 1. Respiratory System—physiology. 2. Respiratory Tract Diseases.
WF 140 M339r]
RC731.M27 1987   616.2   86-33969
ISBN 0-683-05552-6

91 92 93 94   4 5 6 7 8 9 10 11 12 13 14 15

To my parents, Warren and Theresa Marini

Preface to
the Second Edition

In the five years since the initial publication of this book, respiratory medicine has undergone radical change. Apart from rapid advances in understanding that characterize most areas within medicine, the field itself has also redefined its scope, deepening its commitment to the maturing discipline of intensive care. The present-day pulmonologist is often regarded as a subspecialist in critical care, with substantial knowledge of the acute hematologic, gastrointestinal, neurologic, renal, infectious, and cardiovascular problems that were considered outside his/her purview a short time ago.

In view of this expanded scope, a single manual of reasonable length cannot contain even the most basic information appropriate to this subspecialty, no matter how concisely written. Therefore, for the second edition I have elected to prepare two separate volumes, Respiratory Medicine and Critical Care Medicine for the House Officer, which will incorporate topics germane to both pulmonary and nonpulmonary intensive care. In so doing I have been able to expand coverage greatly in both areas.

This edition of Respiratory Medicine retains the orientation of the original volume. Like the first, it is not intended to be a comprehensive review. Rather, the material selected for inclusion provides a basis for approaching the respiratory problems that a physician is most frequently called upon to address, with a concentration on adult inpatient illness. Once again, I have tried to include interesting and practical information that is difficult to find elsewhere, excluding much that is either commonly known or easily accessed in standard sources. Chapter length and depth of treatment vary with my perception of the importance of the topic and the knowledge base of the physician. A great deal of material has been added, including new chapters on Chronic Cough, Disorders of the Ventilatory Pump, Pneumonitis in the Immunosuppressed Host, Restrictive Lung Disease, and Tuberculosis and Fungal Diseases of the Lung. Each of chapters retained from the first edition has been revised and updated and useful literature references added as suggested reading.

John J. Marini

Preface to
the First Edition

Houseofficers work and learn under stressful circumstances. As physicians in training, they have limited experience, and their clinical skills are still developing. Nonetheless, they are charged with primary responsibility for managing important but unfamiliar problems. Decisions must often be made quickly, under pressures arising from precipitous clinical events, too much to do, and too little time.

Apart from an aggressive interest, effective learning in this environment requires knowledgeable colleagues and access to key information. However, an understanding of the best approach to new problems is not easily acquired. Most texts discuss diseases, not problems, and relevant information lies dispersed throughout the medical literature. Some of the most important principles are transmitted verbally and not written at all. As a result, a solid grasp of the approach to many common problems may not be achieved without subspecialty training.

This book attempts to present material that will be useful to nonspecialist physicians caring for hospitalized patients with respiratory disorders and patients requiring noncoronary intensive care. Because each case must be analyzed individually, it stresses principles and guidelines whenever possible, deliberately avoiding the "cookbook" approach. Although it is intended primarily for house officers in internal medicine and surgery, others - particularly non-pulmonary physicians, pulmonary fellows, and nurses who specialize in intensive care - may find it useful.

The text is organized in five sections. Chapters on physiology emphasize principles that guide appropriate management of patients with dyspnea. Chapters dealing with clinical skills describe the common bedside procedures related to the respiratory system and focus on the details of technique that help assure a successful outcome. The ancillary diagnostic methods of radiology and nuclear medicine are briefly discussed in the third section, which attempts to transmit succinctly the information needed for optimal use of these services. Chapters on respiratory therapy and intensive care present detailed information on critical-care topics that demand thorough technical comprehension but are often poorly understood by nonspecialists. In this section particular attention is directed to mechanical ventilation, the use of positive end-expiratory pressure, and the interpretation of wedge pressures. The last section, Clinical Notes, describes salient diagnostic and management features of the respiratory problems that most often require attention in the hospital. Although these discussions are not intended to be comprehensive, sufficient detail is provided to permit a firm grasp of the correct management approach.

Admittedly, this is a rather eclectic sampling. I have selected material for its clinical utility and interest while intentionally omitting much of the basic information that I judge to be well known by most house staff or else readily available in other texts and manuals. I have drawn heavily from my experience as a medical house officer and pulmonary fellow, as well as from conversations with my faculty colleagues at the University of Washington. I am particularly indebted to my friend and associate, Dr. Bruce H. Culver, for his thoughtful review of the manuscript and for my own education in this field.

John J. Marini

Acknowledgment

I would like to acknowledge the invaluable assistance of Brenda F. Plunkett, who conducted library research, prepared the typescript, and otherwise contributed greatly to this work.

MILES

Compliments of Miles Inc. Pharmaceutical Division, Maker of

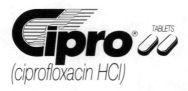

Cipro® *TABLETS*

(ciprofloxacin HCl)

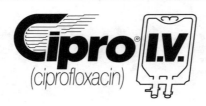

Cipro® **I.V.**

(ciprofloxacin)

Contents

SECTION IV - CLINICAL PROBLEMS

Chapter 1

Thoracic Mechanics

THE RESPIRATORY MUSCLES

Normal Anatomy and Function

Air flows to and from the alveoli driven by differences in pressure between the airway opening and the alveolus. During spontaneous breathing, mouth (atmospheric) pressure is constant, and alveolar pressure fluctuates because of changing pleural pressure and tissue recoil.

During quiet breathing the diaphragm powers inspiration both by displacing the abdominal contents caudally and by actually raising the lower ribs as it contracts. The rib cage musculature is minimally active, with the parasternal and scalene groups routinely developing some degree of tension. Normally exhalation is passive.

When faced with a large ventilatory requirement or with a lung reluctant to move gas because of airway obstruction or parenchymal restriction, accessory muscles of respiration (including external intercostals, sternocleidomastoids, parasternal, and scalene groups) are recruited to aid inhalation. Forceful exhalation is assisted by the internal intercostals and by the abdominal muscles, which contract to thrust the diaphragm upward. The phrenic nerve (C 3-5) innervates the diaphragm, and the spinal nerves (T2-L4) innervate the intercostal and abdominal muscles.

Determinants of Muscle Power

Respiratory muscle strength is determined by muscle bulk, by the chemical environment, and by the intrinsic properties, loading conditions, and geometric orientation of the contractile fibers. Because poor nutrition causes generalized muscle wasting, the mass of the diaphragm relates directly to nutritional status. As overall body weight declines, diaphragmatic mass and strength diminish commensurately. The chemical and hormonal environment of the contracting muscle also influences performance. Concentrations of calcium, magnesium, potassium, phosphate, carbon dioxide, and hydrogen ion are each of demonstrated importance.

Fiber Properties and Orientation

When stimulated at a specific intensity, the force developed by a skeletal muscle fiber diminishes with reductions in resting length. This force-length interaction is a "preloading" phenomenon (similar to the Frank-Starling mechanism) and largely accounts for the dependence of maximal respiratory pressures on lung volume (see p. 6). The force-velocity relationship is another important intrinsic fiber property. Maximal pressures at any muscle length are developed under static, isometric conditions. As the velocity of fiber shortening increases, the force developed diminishes as a die-away exponential function. The geometric orientation of muscle fibers determines whether fiber contraction, however forceful, generates a useful vector in the direction of inspiration or expiration. For example, a flattened diaphragm does not produce an effective inspiratory action because it cannot displace the abdominal contents. Thus, a breathless, hyperinflated patient is triply disadvantaged; not only is the geometry suboptimal for optimal performance, but inspiratory fibers are both shortened and forced to contract rapidly.

Muscular Endurance

The ability of the respiratory muscles to sustain a ventilatory work load is best understood in terms of exertional capability and demand. During unloaded breathing, approximately 50% of the maximum possible ventilation rate (MVV) can be sustained indefinitely. As normal breathing is loaded by obstruction (e.g., asthma) or restriction (e.g., pulmonary edema), higher than normal respiratory pressures must be generated on each breathing cycle. Whether a given level of exertion is well tolerated or overloads the system is determined by the average inspiratory pressure expressed as a fraction of the maximum possible value ($\bar{P}/P_{max}$) and by the fraction of each ventilatory cycle over which this inspiratory pressure must be exerted (T_i/T_{tot}). The product $\bar{P}/P_{max} \times T_i/T_{tot}$ has been termed the "tension-time index" (I_{tt}). Normally $\bar{P}/P_{max}$, T_i/T_{tot}, and I_{tt} average $\simeq$ 0.05, 0.40, and 0.02, respectively. Values of $I_{tt} > 0.20$ invariably lead to fatigue. Lower levels of stress are sufficient to cause fatigue in patients with compromised cardiac function. Once fatigue has been induced by a brief period of stressful breathing, full recovery of endurance may require a lengthy period. Such observations have implications for the degree of support needed during ventilatory crises.

Clinical Signs of Muscle Dysfunction and Fatigue

Increasing tachypnea is the earliest sign of ventilatory distress, particularly when it is accompanied by declining tidal volumes. The abdominal surface normally moves outward as the diaphragm descends. Upon reaching the limits of compensation, paradoxical (inward) inspiratory movement of the diaphragm (abdominal paradox) may be observed in the supine position, a sign of extreme loading or fatigue. The smooth interaction between various respiratory muscle groups may uncouple, causing overt discoordination. Just before total exhaustion is reached, the respiratory rate slows and gasping respirations may be observed.

Neuromuscular Paralysis

When upright, patients with isolated paralysis of both hemidiaphragms can often sustain adequate ventilation by coordinated use of the accessory muscles of inspiration and the abdominal muscles. First, the diaphragm is forced upward as muscles contract to raise abdominal pressure. Then the diaphragm descends, aided by gravity, as muscle relaxation allows abdominal pressure to fall. This mechanism cannot work effectively in the supine position, a circumstance that explains why orthopnea is a prominent symptom of this disorder. Patients with spinal cord injury (quadriplegia) have the converse anatomic problem; the intact diaphragm provides adequate ventilation to meet the normal requirement, but paralysis of expiratory musculature severely limits ventilatory reserve and coughing efficiency.

PRESSURE-VOLUME RELATIONSHIPS

The lung and its thoracic shell occupy an identical volume except when air or fluid separates them. At any specified volume the pressure acting to distend the lung is alveolar pressure minus pleural pressure (transpulmonary pressure, P_{tp}), whereas the pressure across the chest wall is pleural pressure minus atmospheric pressure. The volume of the lung is determined uniquely by the compliance of the lung and the pressure difference acting to distend it (P_{tp}). The lung requires more pressure to achieve than to hold any specified lung volume, a characteristic known as inflation hysteresis.

If compliance and transpulmonary pressure are identical, lung volume is the same. (It does not matter whether the alveolar pressure is 0 and pleural pressure is -5 cmH$_2$O or if alveolar pressure is 25 and pleural pressure is 20.) A similar relationship between distending pressure, compliance, and volume also applies to the chest wall.

When the chest wall muscles are relaxed at end expiration (functional residual capacity, FRC), the tendency of the chest wall to spring outward just balances the tendency of the lung to recoil inward to a smaller volume. Should either the lung or the chest wall become less compliant (as in interstitial fibrosis or obesity, respectively), the pressure-volume curve shifts rightward and flattens, causing FRC to decrease. Conversely, increased lung compliance (as in emphysema) allows a higher resting volume.

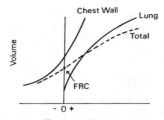

Figure 1.1. Relationship between volume and transmural pressure across the lung (airway pressure minus pleural pressure, expiratory limb), across the relaxed chest wall (pleural pressure minus atmospheric pressure), and across both structures (airway pressure minus atmospheric pressure). At FRC, recoil pressures of lung and chest wall are equal but directly opposed.

PLEURAL PRESSURE

The fraction of any change in alveolar pressure sensed in the pleural space will depend upon the relative compliances of the lung (C_l) and chest wall (C_{cw}). For a given change in alveolar pressure (ΔP_A), the amount transmitted to the pleural space (ΔP_{pl}) will be

$$\Delta P_{pl} = \Delta P_A \times (C_l) / (C_l + C_{cw})$$

An infinitely stiff chest wall would allow no volume change of the lung and complete transmission of a given increment in alveolar pressure to the pleural space. Conversely, an infinitely stiff lung would transmit none of it. Under normal circumstances the lung and chest wall are almost equally compliant throughout the tidal range so that approximately half of any change in alveolar pressure (as when PEEP is applied) registers in the pleural space.

Although clinicians are fond of speaking of pleural pressure as if it were a unique number, pleural pressure varies considerably because of hydrostatic gradients (which at FRC average 0.3 cmH$_2$O per cm of vertical height) and because the pleural space and mediastinum have irregular contours caused by bony and vascular structures. At FRC, average pleural pressure at mid-lung level is negative because the lung is held open at greater than its relaxed volume. Pleural pressure surrounds the heart, the great vessels, and large airways and therefore affects the vascular pressures measured at intrathoracic sites. Relative changes in pleural pressure can be accurately monitored with the use of a balloon manometer positioned in the mid esophagus.

EFFECT OF CHANGES IN LUNG VOLUME

Airway Resistance

Pleural pressure surrounds the largest airways, whereas airways deeper within the lung are tethered open by the recoil forces of the surrounding alveoli.   Hence, as lung volume increases, the diameter of all airways increases, and resistance falls. Conversely, if a normal lung is held at a low resting volume (as in obesity), airway resistance will be relatively high. Because resistance is inversely proportional to the fourth power of airway radius, lung volume can strongly influence its value.

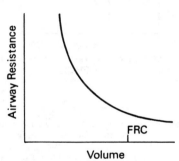

Figure 1.2. Relationship of airway resistance to lung volume. Airway resistance rises markedly as volume decreases below FRC.

In most restrictive diseases of lung tissue (e.g., interstitial fibrosis) the effects of heightened recoil on airway diameter and driving force cause flow rates to be high relative to lung volume.

Pulmonary Vascular Resistance

Raising lung volume has a different effect on the resistance in pulmonary vessels. Although extra-alveolar vessels expand under a tractive force similar to that acting on the airways, capillaries are compressed.   Net pulmonary vascular resistance increases with each increment in lung volume above FRC.

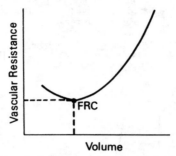

Figure 1.3. Relationship of pulmonary vascular resistance to lung volume. Minimum vascular resistance occurs near FRC.

Muscular Force

Lung volume has an important effect on the maximal force that can be generated by the respiratory system. The magnitude of this force can be quantified by measuring the maximal pressure sustained during airway occlusion. At total lung capacity (TLC), the lung and chest wall exert their highest recoil pressures. More importantly, the muscles of expiration are stretched maximally and hence are able to generate their highest contractile forces. Thus, to be maximally effective, a coughing effort must start from a high lung volume.

The greatest inspiratory pressure can be generated at residual volume, where the muscle fibers of the diaphragm are stretched to a position of maximal mechanical advantage. (This encourages some patients to unintentionally misuse incentive spirometers, which place emphasis on flow rate rather than inhaled volume; they exhale below FRC in order to profit from higher inspiratory muscle efficiency.) Conversely, hyperinflation causes the diaphragm to work less effectively, adding to the sense of dyspnea experienced by patients with chronic obstructive pulmonary disease (COPD).

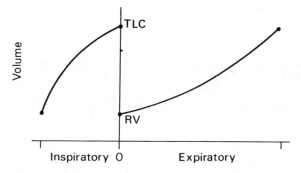

Maximal Pressure

Figure 1.4. Relationship between lung volume and the maximal pressure developed against an occluded airway. Expiratory effort is most effective at high lung volumes; inspiratory effort is best at low lung volumes.

Position and Lung Volume

Position has an important influence on lung volume. Upon assuming a recumbent supine position, FRC normally falls approximately 25-30% from the sitting value, with most of the decrease occurring before the Fowler's (30°) position. This reduction in lung volume occurs because the abdominal contents push the diaphragm cephalad. In either lateral recumbent position, lung volume at FRC is only about 15-20% less than the upright sitting value, because the nondependent (uppermost) lung maintains or increases its resting lung volume. Although positional lung volume changes may be less in patients with diseased lungs, such observations have relevance for the nursing care of postoperative and critically ill patients.

NORMAL PATTERN OF BREATHING

To provide approximately 5 liters of fresh gas per minute to the lungs, the thoracic pump moves a stroke (tidal) volume of 5-7 ml/kg at a frequency of 10-16/minute. At frequent intervals, sighs 2-5 times as large as the normal tidal volume are taken to oppose the natural tendency for dependent alveoli to collapse when ventilated continuously at a normal but monotonous volume. Breath to breath, the end-expiratory lung volume (FRC) changes continuously about a constant average value.

DEAD SPACE

The bronchial, pharyngeal, and nasal passages must be ventilated but do not participate in gas exchange. This anatomic dead space varies with airway caliber and lung volume, averaging roughly 2.2 ml/kg (1 ml/lb) of lean body weight at FRC. Because approximately 50% of this dead space resides in the upper airways, orotracheal intubation and tracheostomy cut anatomic dead space significantly.

In addition to anatomic dead space, some volume of fresh gas reaches alveoli but does not participate in gas exchange because of inadequate perfusion. Part of the increased ventilatory requirement seen after a large pulmonary embolus results from this mechanism. Taken together, anatomic and alveolar dead space constitute the physiological dead space, i.e., the volume of gas moved during each tidal breath that does not participate in gas exchange. The fraction of each tidal breath wasted in this fashion, V_D/V_T, can be accurately approximated by the formula:

$$V_D/V_T = (PaCO_2 - P_ECO_2)/PaCO_2$$

where $PaCO_2$ and P_ECO_2 are the partial pressures of CO_2 in arterial blood and mixed expired gas, respectively. V_D/V_T increases with age. During exercise, V_D/V_T may fall to 20% or less, owing both to larger tidal breaths and to better perfusion throughout the lung. At very low tidal volumes, V_D/V_T rises to a high value because anatomic dead space does not decrease proportionately. (Nonetheless, even at tidal volumes theoretically smaller than the anatomic dead space value, some alveolar gas exchange does occur, as exemplified by high-frequency ventilation.)

FLOW LIMITATION

The rate of airflow depends upon the pressure difference driving flow and airway resistance: flow = (driving pressure)/(resistance). Flow rates during exhalation are volume dependent because the airway caliber and the recoil pressure driving gas flow increase progressively with lung volume.

Normally, the major site of flow resistance resides in the nasal passages, larynx, and uppermost tracheal airway. During quiet tidal breathing the average pleural pressure surrounding the large airways varies from about

-2 cmH$_2$O to -10 cmH$_2$O, never reaching a positive value relative to intraluminal pressure. As a result there are no compressive forces tending to narrow the airway during passive exhalation.

Forceful efforts to exhale raise pleural pressure to positive values. Increased pleural pressure adds to lung recoil, boosting alveolar pressure and increasing the pressure available to drive gas flow. However, because pressure within the airway declines progressively as the airway opening is approached, positive pleural pressure simultaneously acts to narrow the compressible intrathoracic airway.

Passive Exhalation	Moderate Effort	Maximal Effort

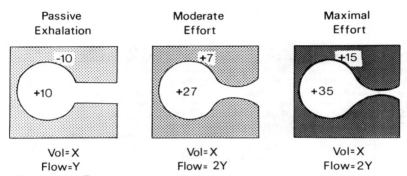

Vol= X	Vol= X	Vol= X
Flow=Y	Flow= 2Y	Flow= 2Y

Figure 1.5. Effect of increasing effort on expiratory flow rate at the same lung volume. Increasing expiratory force raises alveolar driving pressure but tends also to compress intrathoracic airways. Beyond a moderately forceful effort, these effects offset each other, and rate of airflow does not increase.

At efforts greater than 2/3 of maximum, each additional increment of pleural pressure narrows the airway sufficiently to offset the increment in alveolar pressure. Flow is then effort independent and remains so at smaller lung volumes, so long as forceful effort is sustained. The point within the airway where pleural pressure and intraluminal pressure are equal ("the equal pressure point") determines where critical narrowing occurs. In normals it resides in the trachea or main bronchi at high lung volumes and migrates toward the alveolus as forced expiration proceeds. Maximal flows in the very first part of exhalation - the first 20% - still depend upon effort. At smaller volumes, maximal flow is determined only by the recoil pressure of the lung and the resistance of the airway segment upstream of the equal pressure point.

Reproducibility stemming from effort independence is the major reason why indices of forced spirometry (such as FEV_1) enjoy popularity as a method of evaluating airflow obstruction. Peak flow rate, which occurs before 25% of the vital capacity has been exhaled, and all inspiratory flow rates are effort dependent and therefore less reproducible. Many patients with airflow obstruction are flow limited throughout much of the ventilatory cycle, even under optimal conditions. Indeed, some patients with emphysema have such collapsible airways that flow rates demonstrate negative effort dependence; i.e., flow rates worsen with increasing effort. Presumably this helps account for the practice of pursed-lip breathing among patients who are so severely limited by their disease that they must utilize optimal rates of exhalation continuously.

WORK OF BREATHING

In moving gas to and from the alveoli, energy must be expended primarily against frictional and elastic forces. As ventilation requirement increases, the total work of breathing rises disproportionately; gas must be moved at a greater rate of speed, and increased tidal volumes extract a greater energy cost. The major portion of frictional resistance arises from collisions of gas molecules with the surfaces of the airway. Work done against friction depends strongly upon airway size, increasing rapidly as airway caliber narrows. For this reason frictional work varies inversely with lung volume, which helps determine luminal diameter. When airways are narrowed by obstructive disease, a relatively small increase in resting lung volume can substantially reduce the work dissipated against frictional forces.

The elastic forces that oppose ventilation originate within the lung parenchyma and chest wall. Elastic recoil increases in a nearly linear fashion with lung volume throughout the physiologic range. Diseases such as interstitial fibrosis and obesity may dramatically increase the effort required to distend the lung.

When total work done against combined frictional and elastic forces is plotted against lung volume, the minimum value normally occurs near FRC. Patients with airflow obstruction reduce their work if they breathe at a relatively high lung volume, since frictional work may fall dramatically as lung volume increases. Conversely, patients with restrictive parenchymal lung disease may perform less total work at lower lung volumes, as the reduction in elastic work outstrips the increase in frictional work.

Under normal circumstances, FRC and breathing frequency are set to minimize the total work of breathing. At a specified level of ventilation, increasing tidal volume increases the work done against elastic forces and reduces frictional pressure losses. The optimal breathing pattern varies with lung pathophysiology. For example, in cases of advanced airflow obstruction, acceptable ventilation may require that the patient maintain a high lung volume in order to take advantage of the flow rates achievable at that level. (At a lower FRC, expiratory flow is too slow to allow adequate alveolar ventilation.) For similar reasons, a larger tidal volume and slower breathing frequency are most energetically efficient, even if not always adopted.

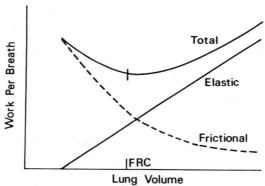

Figure 1.6. Relationship of lung volume and work done against elastic and frictional forces. Normally, total work of breathing is minimized at a lung volume near FRC.

Clinical Measurement of the Work of Breathing

Two methods for estimating the ventilatory work load have been used successfully in the laboratory setting: determination of oxygen consumption ($\dot{V}O_2$) before and after a ventilatory stress and direct measurement of the work done in effecting a volume change. Technical obstacles, however, have prevented the widespread application of these methods to clinical problems. $\dot{V}O_2$ changes rapidly and is difficult to measure with acceptable accuracy in patients inspiring high oxygen fractions. On the other hand, the mechanical work (W) performed across a passive structure, such as the lung, can be accurately quantified as the integral of its inflating pressure (P) and flow ($\dot{V}$): $W = \int P\dot{V}dt$. For the lung, P is the difference between airway and pleural pressures. Integration can be accomplished electronically or by measuring the area enclosed beneath a display of P against inspired volume, the time integral of airflow. For patients receiving mechanical ventilation, the work of passive chest inflation can be quantified from bedside estimation of the mean change in airway pressure required to deliver tidal volume at the selected rate of airflow.

SUGGESTED READINGS

1.   Derenne JP, Macklem PT, Roussos C.   The respiratory muscles: mechanics control and pathophysiology.   Am. Rev. Respir. Dis. 1978;118:119-33,373-90,581-601.

2.   Fishman AP, Macklem PT, Mead J, eds. Mechanics of Breathing (Volume 3 of the Respiratory System, Section 3). In: Handbook of Physiology. Bethesda, MD: American Physiological Society, 1986.

3.   Marini JJ, et al. Influence of head-dependent positions on lung volume and oxygen saturation in chronic air-flow obstruction. Am. Rev. Respir. Dis. 1984;129:101-05.

4.   Marini JJ, Rodriguez RM, Lamb V. Bedside estimation of the inspiratory work of breathing during mechanical ventilation. Chest 1986;89:56-63.

5.   Marini JJ, Rodriguez RM, Lamb V. The inspiratory workload of patient-initiated mechanical ventilation. Am. Rev. Respir. Dis. 1986;134:902-09.

6.   Murray JF. The Normal Lung. 2nd ed. Philadelphia: WB Saunders, 1986.

7.   Otis AB. The work of breathing. Phys. Rev. 1954;34:449-58.

8.   Roussos C, Macklem PT. The respiratory muscles. N. Engl. J. Med. 1982;307:786-97.

Chapter 2

Ventilation-Perfusion Relationships

DISTRIBUTION OF VENTILATION AND PERFUSION

Ventilation ($\dot{V}$)

Alveoli contiguous to the pleura are kept open by a positive distending pressure (alveolar-pleural). At the same horizontal level, a net pressure nearly equal to pleural pressure surrounds an alveolus deep within the lung parenchyma. This is due to the phenomenon of interdependence, which bridges each alveolar wall with its immediate and distant neighbors.

Although the alveolar distending pressures across a given horizontal slice of the lung are similar, the vertical gradient of pleural pressure (approximately 0.3 cmH$_2$O/vertical cm at FRC) causes a more negative pleural pressure at the apex of the upright lung than at the base. Consequently, apical alveoli and airways are larger at FRC than their basilar counterparts. However, the thorax has an irregular shape, and as pleural pressure falls during inhalation, it does so unevenly; pressure falls most in the dependent regions closest to the diaphragm. This larger pressure swing, together with the fact that smaller alveoli are more compliant than larger ones, causes the lung bases to ventilate better than the apices. The same principles hold in the supine, prone, and lateral positions: uppermost lung regions are held more widely open, but the dependent lung regions are better ventilated during spontaneous breathing - a good rationale for turning bedridden patients frequently from side to side.

Perfusion ($\dot{Q}$)

The relationship of ventilation to dependency is fortunate, considering that the distribution of blood flow follows a similar rule. Because of its low resistance, the normal pulmonary circulation is a low-pressure circuit, with resting pressures in the central pulmonary arteries averaging approximately 25/10 mmHg (mean 15 mmHg). Pulmonary venous pressure is similar to that of the left atrium, oscillating between 3 and 10 mmHg with the cardiac cycle. Because the apices lie at least 10 centimeters above the hilae in the upright position, capillaries there must wink open and closed. However, at the bases, hydrostatic pressure adds to intraluminal pressure so that vessels in dependent regions remain relatively dilated, and the driving pressure for flow there is relatively high. Hence, perfusion improves markedly from apex to base. This helps explain why emboli localize to the lower lobes and why collapse of air spaces at the base can cause profound hypoxemia, whereas upper lobe atelectasis seldom does. Given a patient with unilateral parenchymal disease and a choice of placing the patient in either lateral position to improve gas exchange, the "good" lung should be placed dependent for two reasons: the "good" lung will receive a higher percentage of total ventilation and perfusion, and the "bad" lung will be subjected to higher distending pressures.

Although dependency causes both ventilation and perfusion per unit volume to increase, the effect on perfusion is more striking. The ratio of ventilation to perfusion, therefore, is highest at the apex and lowest at the base.

REGULATION OF REGIONAL PERFUSION

Regional perfusion is governed by the pressure driving flow and the impedance to fluid movement through the vascular network. Normally resistance is partitioned more evenly along the pulmonary vascular channel than it is in the systemic circulation. The overall resistance of the pulmonary vascular bed is not fixed. At any moment the number of channels available to carry flow will vary with gravitational and mechanical stresses.

Hydrostatics

Blood flow through a lung region is influenced by the relationship between alveolar pressure and pulmonary arterial and venous pressures. If alveolar pressure (P_A) exceeds arterial pressure (P_a), alveolar capillaries will pinch closed and no blood will flow. If P_A is less than P_a but exceeds venous pressure (P_v), flow through the region will be driven by the difference between P_a and P_A (not P_v). If P_v exceeds P_A, flow will be governed by the arterial-venous pressure difference and independent of alveolar pressure. At the very base of the lung, interstitial pressure (P_i) is high relative to P_A or P_v, and flow is governed by the $P_a - P_i$ difference. Zones reflecting each of these conditions can be identified during tidal breathing. The influence of alveolar pressure on capillary patency is particularly important to consider when high levels of positive end-expiratory pressure are applied to the airway, raising P_A relative to P_v. When P_A exceeds P_v, balloon-occlusion pulmonary artery (wedge) pressure will reflect alveolar, not pulmonary venous pressure (see p. 161).

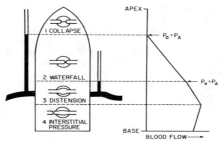

Figure 2.1. Schematic representation of the four zones of the lung in which different hemodynamic conditions govern blood flow. Alveolar pressure (P_A) is assumed to be 0; the heights of the black columns on the left and right of the lung represent the magnitude of pulmonary arterial and venous pressures, respectively. (Adapted from Reference 4).

Capillary Recruitment

At a specified lung volume, pulmonary vascular resistance falls as flow increases. Rising pulmonary arterial pressure recruits previously unperfused capillaries so that a fivefold increase in cardiac output during exercise results in a smaller than twofold increase in mean pulmonary artery pressure. Ventilation to perfusion matchup also becomes more uniform under these conditions. In a patient with a partially obliterated pulmonary vascular bed (e.g., emphysema or interstitial fibrosis), few capillaries may remain to be recruited at rest. Under this condition, even modest increments in cardiac output or pulmonary vascular resistance cause pulmonary artery pressure to increase dramatically.

Active Vasoconstriction

Apart from the effect of capillary recruitment, pulmonary blood flow can be regionally controlled by active constriction of vascular smooth muscle. If vascular smooth muscle hypertrophies due to chronic hypertension, response to vasoconstricting stimuli may be exaggerated. Alveolar hypoxia exerts by far the most important influence on local vasoconstriction. Normally, this property serves a useful purpose, diverting blood away from alveoli that are poorly ventilated. However, acting against the background of a restricted capillary bed, widespread hypoxic vasoconstriction may cause excessive pulmonary artery pressure and precipitate acute right ventricular failure, as in decompensated COPD. Acidemia is a weaker stimulus to pulmonary artery vasoconstriction but adds to the effect of alveolar hypoxia.

Other stimuli can influence vasomotor tone. Hypertonic fluids, such as angiographic contrast media, can precipitate a striking vasoconstrictor response. This may be an important mechanism causing sudden death in patients with pulmonary hypertension during angiographic studies. Vasoactive substances, such as serotonin, histamine, and certain prostaglandins, also produce notable vasoconstriction, and their effects may vary from site to site along the arteriovenous pathway. Alpha-adrenergic vasopressors (e.g., levarterenol) cause little response. Unfortunately, few available drugs produce potent vasodilatation. However, aminophylline, isoproterenol, tolazoline, hydralazine, and nifedepine are pulmonary vasodilators. Acetylcholine, although active, has associated adverse side effects that prevent its use.

REGULATION OF REGIONAL VENTILATION

Ventilation to a given lung region depends not only on the stress applied but also on the regional compliance of that unit and the resistance it offers to air entry. The product of resistance and compliance is known as the "time constant," RC, by analogy with an electrical oscillator. A region with a low time constant (e.g., a stiff unit with open conducting airway) will fill and empty rapidly and be relatively well ventilated for the amount of stress applied, compared to immediate neighbors having longer time constants. Because diseased lungs have regions of varied time constants, the distribution of ventilation tends to become progressively uneven the faster pressure changes occur.

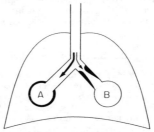

Figure 2.2. Schematic diagram of two lung units with varying time constants (τ = RC). Unit A is a low-compliance unit served by a widely patent bronchus, whereas unit B is a normally compliant unit whose airflow is impeded. Because τ_A is shorter than τ_B, unit A will be better ventilated for an equivalent stress.

Healthy lungs depend upon bronchial smooth muscle to regulate the resistance of local units. Contraction of bronchial smooth muscle is influenced by multiple autonomic and biochemical stimuli, many of which are only now being defined. Both beta-sympathetic and parasympathetic nerves innervate bronchial smooth muscle. The importance of alpha-receptor stimulation has been difficult to demonstrate in man. Vagal fibers distribute throughout the tracheobronchial tree, whereas sympathetics tend to concentrate in small airways. The vagus is tonically active, even under normal resting conditions. Irritating stimuli, such as smoke, chemical vapors, and cold air, can amplify its action, triggering mild generalized bronchoconstriction. Carbon dioxide bronchodilates, whereas hypocarbia bronchoconstricts. Diminished CO_2 concentration and resulting bronchoconstriction may partially explain the ventilation defects occasionally seen in the region of a pulmonary embolus. Hypoxemia, acidosis, and altered tonicity of the bronchial mucosa may also cause mild bronchoconstriction.

Many circulating agents affect bronchial tone. Epinephrine and other catecholamines, which stimulate beta-receptors, bronchodilate, as do cholinergic blockers, certain prostaglandins, and theophylline derivatives. Histamine, certain leukotrienes, and thromboxanes (prostaglandin metabolites) tend to bronchoconstrict.

SUGGESTED READINGS

1. Comroe JH Jr, et al. The Lung, 2nd ed. Chicago: Yearbook Medical Publishers, 1962;27-110.

2. Murray JF. The Normal Lung, 2nd ed. Philadelphia: WB Saunders, 1986.

3. Nunn JF. Applied Respiratory Physiology, 2nd ed. Boston: Butterworths, 1977;274-309.

4. West JB. Ventilation: Blood Flow and Gas Exchange, 2nd ed. Oxford: Blackwell, 1970.

Chapter 3

Gas Exchange and Transport

ALVEOLAR GAS EXCHANGE

Respiratory Quotient

The primary function of ventilation is to allow the exchange of CO_2 generated in body tissues for O_2 available in the inspired gas. For a resting adult of average size, approximately 250 ml of O_2 are consumed by the tissues per minute ($\dot{V}O_2$) while 200 ml of CO_2 are generated ($\dot{V}CO_2$), a respiratory "quotient" (RQ = $\dot{V}CO_2/\dot{V}O_2$) of 0.8. Over a long period of time the ratio of gases exchanged with the atmosphere, R, must equal RQ. Transiently, however, R may exceed or be less than RQ, as during brief periods of hyper- or hypoventilation. Important increases in RQ can occur with a shift to a high-carbohydrate diet, with refeeding after a period of starvation, and with the development of certain metabolically stressful conditions (e.g., sepsis).

Alveolar Gas Equation

Gases move between the blood and alveolar spaces by diffusion from areas of high partial pressure to those with lower partial pressure. As fresh gas is inspired at ambient barometric pressure, it is warmed to body temperature and fully humidified before it reaches the main carina. At saturation, the partial pressure exerted by water vapor at 37° is 47 mmHg, independent of barometric pressure. Thus, $P_iO_2 = F_iO_2 (P_B - 47)$, where P_iO_2 is the partial pressure of oxygen in the central airways, F_iO_2 is the fraction of oxygen in the inspired gas mixture, and P_B is barometric pressure (mmHg). P_B falls with altitude, relatively quickly at elevations close to sea level (P_B is approximately 520 mmHg at 10,000 feet).

In the steady state the partial pressure of oxygen at the alveolar level, P_AO_2, can be calculated from the simplified alveolar gas equation, which is based on the principle of conservation of mass:

$$P_AO_2 = P_iO_2 - (P_ACO_2)/R$$

(P_ACO_2 and the partial pressure of CO_2 in arterial blood, or $PaCO_2$, remain nearly equivalent, even in disease, so that $PaCO_2$ is usually measured and substituted.) Transient episodes of hyperventilation and breath-holding can result in oxygen tensions that are considerably higher or lower than the predicted values.

Alveolar-Arterial Oxygen Tension Difference

The alveolar gas equation is worth remembering because the difference between calculated P_AO_2 and measured PaO_2 (known variously as the (A-a) PO_2 difference, the (A-a)DO_2, or the A-a gradient) provides a measure of the efficiency of gas exchange between the alveolus and the arterial blood. The normal (A-a)DO_2 increases with F_iO_2, with age, and with body position. For a healthy, young person at sea level, (A-a)DO_2 is approximately 10 mmHg while breathing air and 100 mmHg while breathing 100% oxygen. Hyper- and hypoventilation do not affect it. The (A-a)DO_2 is a useful index when monitoring patients who require supplemental oxygen, but is F_iO_2 dependent. The PaO_2/P_AO_2 ratio is less affected by differences in inspired oxygen concentration.

Causes of Arterial Hypoxemia

Arterial oxygen content may fall due to one of six mechanisms: (1) inhalation of a hypoxic gas mixture, (2) hypoventilation, (3) impaired diffusion of oxygen from alveolar space to pulmonary capillary, (4) ventilation/perfusion ($\dot{V}/\dot{Q}$) mismatching, (5) shunting of venous blood past alveolar capillaries, (6) admixture of abnormally desaturated systemic venous blood. A decrease in the inspired fraction of oxygen, as at high altitude, will cause hypoxemia for obvious reasons. In the steady state, hypoventilation will cause alveolar PO_2 to fall as oxygen is consumed but not replenished at normal rates, in accordance with the alveolar gas equation. Under certain conditions, impaired diffusion of oxygen can result in incomplete equilibration of gas tensions in the alveolus and the pulmonary capillary. Increased distance for diffusion between alveolus and erythrocyte, decreased partial pressure gradient driving diffusion, and shortened transit time of the red cell through the capillary all adversely influence diffusion. Under ordinary circumstances, however, none of these factors acting in isolation slows equilibration sufficiently to allow desaturation of end-capillary blood. Nonetheless, a combination of adverse influences may cause enough impairment of diffusion to contribute to hypoxemia (e.g., diffusion impairment probably contributes to the hypoxemia of a person with interstitial fibrosis during exercise).

$\dot{V}/\dot{Q}$ Mismatching

Regional mismatching of ventilation to perfusion is perhaps the most frequent cause of clinically important desaturation (e.g., COPD). The problem is distributional. When the entire lung is considered, it is not the ratio of minute ventilation relative to pulmonary blood flow that determines whether hypoxemia occurs but rather whether ventilation and perfusion distribute appropriately. (For example, one lung could receive all ventilation and the other all perfusion for an overall $\dot{V}/\dot{Q}$ ratio of 1.0.) Units that are relatively poorly ventilated in relation to their perfusion cause desaturation; high $\dot{V}/\dot{Q}$ units contribute to physiologic dead space (wasted ventilation) but not to hypoxemia. Unfortunately, overventilating some units to compensate for others that are underventilated keeps $PaCO_2$, but not PaO_2, at the proper level. Aliquots of blood exiting from different lung units mix gas <u>contents,</u> not partial pressures. Because the blood content of CO_2 relates linearly to alveolar ventilation in the physiologic range, a unit with good ventilation can compensate for an underventilated unit. However, at normal barometric pressure, little more oxygen can be loaded onto blood with already saturated hemoglobin, no matter how high the oxygen tension in the overventilated alveolus may rise (see p. 23). Hence, when equal aliquots of blood from well- and poorly ventilated units mix their contents, the resulting blood will have an O_2 content halfway between them but a PaO_2 only slightly higher than that of the low $\dot{V}/\dot{Q}$ unit.

Increasing the inspired fraction of oxygen will cause arterial hypoxemia to reverse impressively, as the alveolar oxygen partial pressure of even poorly ventilated units climbs high enough to achieve saturation. After breathing 100% oxygen for a sufficient period of time, only those units that are totally or almost totally unventilated will contribute to hypoxemia.

Shunt

Hypoventilation, impaired diffusion, and $\dot{V}/\dot{Q}$ mismatching respond to supplemental oxygen. Units that are totally unventilated are unresponsive to oxygen therapy and contribute to intrapulmonary shunt. Shunt can also be intracardiac, as in cyanotic (right to left) congenital heart disease or can result from passage of blood through abnormal vascular channels within the lung, as with pulmonary arteriovenous communications. If the patient is given oxygen ($F_iO_2 = 1.0$) for fifteen minutes, the percentage of blood flow being shunted can be calculated from the formula:

$$Q_s/Q_t = (C_cO_2 - C_aO_2)/(C_cO_2 - C_{\bar{v}}O_2) \times 100$$

where C denotes content and the subscripts c, a, and v denote end-pulmonary capillary, arterial, and mixed venous, respectively. End-capillary PO_2 is assumed to equal alveolar oxygen tension, which in turn is calculated from the simplified alveolar gas equation. (Although it is best to measure mixed venous oxygen content directly, stable patients with presumed normal cardiac output, oxygen consumption, and hemoglobin can reasonably be estimated to have a normal $C_{\bar{v}}O_2$ so long as arterial blood is near full saturation.) For a patient breathing pure oxygen, shunt fractions less than 25% can be estimated rapidly by dividing the A-a difference ($670 - PaO_2$) by 20 (again with the proviso that mixed venous oxygen content is normal).

At inspired oxygen fractions less than 1.0, true shunt cannot be reliably estimated by an analysis of oxygen contents, but "venous admixture" or "physiological shunt" can. Although $\dot{V}/\dot{Q}$ mismatch as well as true shunt may contribute to a lower than normal PaO_2, any desaturation can be considered as if it all originated from true shunt units. To calculate venous admixture, C_cO_2 in the shunt formula is calculated from the ideal P_AO_2 existing at that particular inspired fraction of oxygen. At the bedside, an imprecise but commonly used indicator of gas exchange is the PaO_2/F_iO_2 ratio (the "P to F" ratio). In healthy adults, this ratio exceeds 400, independently of the F_iO_2.

As the percentage of true shunt rises, supplemental oxygen becomes progressively less effective in raising PaO_2. When true shunt fraction exceeds 25%, little benefit accrues from raising F_iO_2 above 0.5, but the risk of O_2 toxicity escalates and the P/F ratio loses sensitivity. Hence, F_iO_2 can frequently be lowered out of a dangerous range without changing PaO_2 markedly.

However, if venous admixture is due primarily to $\dot{V}/\dot{Q}$ mismatching, the response to raising F_iO_2 will depend on whether most admixture arises from units with nearly normal, moderately low, or very low $\dot{V}/\dot{Q}$ ratios. If hypoxemia is caused by very low $\dot{V}/\dot{Q}$ (but not shunt) units, little improvement may occur until the oxygen fraction approaches 1.0, at which level PaO_2 rises abruptly.

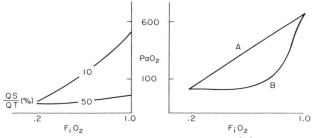

Figure 3.1. The effect of true shunt (QS/QT) and $\dot{V}/\dot{Q}$ mismatching on the relationship between PaO_2 and F_iO_2. Hypoxemia caused by true shunt (left panel) is refractory to supplemental oxygen once QS/QT exceeds 25%. A similar degree of hypoxemia responds to supplemental oxygen if caused by $\dot{V}/\dot{Q}$ mismatching (right panel). However, the F_iO_2 needed depends upon whether hypoxemia is caused by an extensive number of units with mildly abnormal $\dot{V}/\dot{Q}$ mismatch (A) or by a smaller number with very low $\dot{V}/\dot{Q}$ ratios (B).

Admixture of Abnormally Desaturated Venous Blood

Admixture of abnormally desaturated venous blood is a potentially important mechanism acting to lower PaO_2 in patients with impaired pulmonary gas exchange and reduced cardiac output. Oxygen content of venous blood is determined by the interplay between oxygen consumption and oxygen delivery:

$$O_2 \text{ consumption} = (\text{cardiac output}) \times (C_aO_2 - C_{\bar{v}}O_2)$$

Oxygen delivery will be impaired if arterial saturation falls without a compensatory increase in tissue perfusion or if tissue perfusion falls. In the first instance, the peripheral tissues will strip the usual amount of oxygen from an already desaturated hemoglobin molecule, and the resulting venous O_2 content will drop, provided that O_2 consumption remains unchanged. In the second instance, venous O_2 content will fall as an abnormal amount of oxygen is removed from each volume of sluggishly passing blood. Without a compensatory increase in tissue perfusion, anemia can also cause reductions in oxygen delivery, and mixed venous oxygen tension and content.

If all returning venous blood goes to well-ventilated alveoli, abnormally desaturated venous blood presents no problem; blood exiting from the lung will be fully saturated. However, if significant venous admixture exists, a decline in $C_{\bar{v}}O_2$ can translate into arterial desaturation if the shunt fraction remains unchanged. When lung parenchymal disease develops, patients with limited cardiac reserve are those in greatest jeopardy for serious desaturation by this mechanism. Even with stable lung parenchymal disease, serious arterial desaturation can occur if cardiac output falls. Thus, in many intensive care patients, PaO_2 fluctuates considerably, independent of changes in the lungs. Fortunately, shunt fraction tends to decrease when mixed venous oxygen tension falls, presumably because of hypoxic pulmonary vasoconstriction.

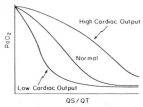

Figure 3.2. Effect of cardiac output on arterial oxygen tension (F_iO_2 constant) for various degrees of venous admixture (QS/QT). As oxygen delivery falls, systemic venous blood desaturates abnormally, causing lower arterial O_2 tension when admixed.

GAS TRANSPORT AND STORAGE

O_2 Carriage

In blood, hemoglobin binds the vast majority of oxygen, and   the remaining small fraction is dissolved in plasma.   The oxyhemoglobin dissociation relationship is curvilinear, with the knee of the curve at approximately 60 mmHg under normal conditions.

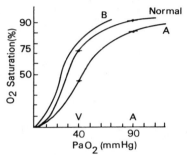

Figure 3.3. Relationship of oxyhemoglobin saturation to partial pressure of oxygen (PaO_2). At oxygen tensions below 60 mmHg, saturation falls abruptly. Acidosis and fever (A) shift the curve rightward, causing a greater saturation difference between arterial (A) and venous (V) blood. Because blood oxygen content parallels oxyhemoglobin saturation, this shift facilitates delivery of oxygen to tissues. Alkalosis and hypothermia (B) have the opposite effect.

Acidosis, increased temperature, raised $PaCO_2$, and increased erythrocyte 2-3 DPG shift the curve rightward, mildly hampering loading at the alveolus but facilitating unloading of oxygen at the low PO_2 of tissue. At sea level, PaO_2 is age dependent, varying from approximately 100 mmHg at age 20 to 80 mmHg at age 80. Because hemoglobin binding is 85-90 percent complete at a partial pressure of 60 mmHg, that level of PaO_2 is commonly agreed to represent adequate oxygen loading and is used as a benchmark value for clinical purposes. The volume (ml) of oxygen carried in a 100-ml aliquot of blood can be calculated from the formula:

$$CaO_2 = .0139 \text{ (Hgb)(\% Sat)} + 0.003 \text{ (}PaO_2\text{)}$$

where Hgb = hemoglobin (grams/100 ml blood) and % Sat = percentage of hemoglobin saturation. At normal levels of circulating hemoglobin, raising PaO_2 tenfold raises oxygen-carrying capacity a scant 12.5%. Yet, in certain settings where the oxygen-carrying capacity of hemoglobin is decreased (e.g., carbon monoxide intoxication or severe anemia) the extra volume of dissolved oxygen gained by breathing pure oxygen may, percentagewise, greatly improve O_2 delivery.

At normal rates of oxygen consumption and delivery, mixed venous blood of normal hemoglobin content has a PO_2 of 40 mmHg, a saturation of 75%, and an oxygen content of 15 ml O_2 per 100 ml of blood. The content difference between simultaneous arterial and mixed venous samples, the (a-v)O_2 difference, averages 5 gm per 100 ml under normal circumstances. However, this difference widens when O_2 consumption is disproportionate to the rate of O_2 delivery to the tissues, as commonly occurs in states of low cardiac output and anemia. Conversely, the (a-v)O_2 difference will be inappropriately narrow if there are functional arteriovenous shunts in peripheral tissues (e.g., cirrhosis, sepsis) or if cardiac output is too high for the metabolic demand.

CO_2 Carriage

Carbon dioxide is carried in the blood in three forms. The small proportion physically dissolved in plasma contributes little to CO_2 exchange between venous blood and the alveolus (about 10% of the total). CO_2 is also bound to blood proteins (mainly hemoglobin), more avidly by venous than by arterial blood. Approximately 30% of the CO_2 delivered to the alveolus is released from these "carbamino" compounds. Quantitatively, the majority of CO_2 carried in blood takes the form of bicarbonate ion stored in the red blood cell. Erythrocytic carbonic anhydrase speeds its conversion to CO_2 as it reaches the alveolus. In this way bicarbonate transports approximately 60% of the total CO_2 exchanged.

Stores of O_2 and CO_2

Exclusive of the gas volume of the lungs, total body tissue stores of oxygen are small, scarcely more than one liter in all. In addition, a considerable proportion of O_2 stores is not available to the tissues without unacceptable reductions in PO_2 and the gradient for diffusion of oxygen at the tissue level. Following sudden cessation of the circulation, supplies are rapidly exhausted, and irreversible damage to vital organs occurs within minutes. When breathing air the lungs act as a reservoir, storing approximately 500 ml of oxygen. Hence, PaO_2 and tissue tensions of oxygen fall more slowly during apnea than during circulatory arrest. (For this reason, attempts to maintain adequate forward blood flow must not be interrupted during resuscitation.) When filled with pure oxygen rather than air, the capacity of the lung reservoir is increased fivefold, and the duration of apnea before hypoxemia occurs is prolonged threefold or longer.

Breathing oxygen does little to increase storage in blood and other body tissues, and P_AO_2 falls precipitously on returning to breathing room air. Thus, "preoxygenating" a patient before endotracheal suction is ineffective if more than a few seconds elapse and is maximally effective if oxygen is continued up until the time that suction is applied. Similar considerations apply during endotracheal intubation. If a tube cannot be placed quickly, the effort should not be prolonged.

By comparison with O_2 stores, body stores of carbon dioxide are enormous, on the order of 100 times as great. As a result, it takes much longer for CO_2 to find its steady-state level after a step change in ventilation. Interestingly, $PaCO_2$ more rapidly achieves the steady-state value following a step increase in ventilation than following a step decrease. Following an exponential curve, the $PaCO_2$ achieves its final value within 10-15 minutes after an increase, but not for a half hour or more following a decrease. These rules of thumb are helpful when deciding the time for arterial blood gas sampling during weaning efforts or when adjusting ventilator settings.

SUGGESTED READINGS

1. Comroe JH. Transport of oxygen (Chapter 14) and Transport of carbon dioxide (Chapter 15). In: Physiology of Respiration (2nd ed.). Chicago: Yearbook Medical Publishers, 1974:183-96 and 201-19.

2. Klocke RA. Arterial blood gases (Chapter 6). In: Baum GL and Wolinsky E, eds. Textbook of Pulmonary Diseases (3rd ed.). Boston: Little Brown, 1983:117-43.

3. Nunn JF. Carbon dioxide (Chapter 11) and Oxygen (Chapter 12). In: Applied Respiratory Physiology (2nd ed.). Boston: Butterworths, 1977:334-444.

4. West JB, Wagner PD. Pulmonary gas exchange. In: West JB, ed. Bioengineering Aspects of the Lung. New York: Marcel Dekker, 1977:361-458.

Chapter 4

Consequences of Altered
PaO₂, PaCO₂, pH

OXYGEN

Hypoxemia

   Arterial blood must deliver enough oxygen to satisfy tissue needs. This requires a tension sufficient to drive O_2 at the required rate to mitochondria at the tissue cores most distant from the capillary. Therefore, two characteristics of arterial oxygenation are important: the quantity of oxygen delivered per unit time ($\dot{Q}$ x CaO_2) and the arterial partial pressure of oxygen (PaO_2).

   Whether a fall in arterial oxygen tension is tolerated well or poorly depends not only upon the extent of desaturation but also upon compensatory mechanisms and the sensitivity of the vital organs to hypoxic stress. Apart from increased oxygen extraction, the major mechanisms of compensation are increased cardiac output, improved perfusion of vital tissues (due to capillary recruitment and changes in distribution of resistance), and red cell manufacture erythrocytosis. Other adaptations, such as improved unloading of oxygen by tissue acidosis and increased anaerobic metabolism, assume importance when failure of the primary methods calls them into action (as during maximal exercise or circulatory arrest). When compensatory reserves are exhausted, the metabolic rate of oxygen consumption ($\dot{V}O_2$) must fall. $\dot{V}O_2$ becomes "delivery dependent" at that point.

   If an individual without cardiac limitation or anemia is made mildly hypoxic over a short period of time, no important effect will be noted until PaO_2 falls below 50-60 mmHg. At that level, malaise, lightheadedness, mild nausea, vertigo, impaired judgment, and incoordination are generally the first symptoms noted, reflecting the extreme sensitivity of cerebral tissue to hypoxia. Although minute ventilation increases, little dyspnea develops unless hyperpnea uncovers underlying mechanical lung problems, as in COPD. Confusion resembling alcohol intoxication appears as PaO_2 falls into the 35-50 mmHg range, especially in older individuals with ischemic cerebrovascular disease. Heart rhythm disturbances also develop. Between 25 and 35 mmHg, renal blood flow decreases and urine output slows. Lactic acidosis appears at this level, even with normal cardiac function. The patient becomes lethargic or obtunded and minute ventilation is maximal. At approximately 25 mmHg the normal individual loses consciousness, and below that tension minute ventilation falls due to depression of the respiratory center.

This sequence of events will be shifted to occur at progressively higher levels of oxygen tension if any of the major compensatory mechanisms for hypoxemia is defective. Even mild decreases in oxygen tension are poorly tolerated by an anemic patient with impaired cardiac output or coronary insufficiency. In addition, critically ill patients may have impaired autonomic control of perfusion distribution, due either to endogenous pathology (e.g., sepsis) or to vasopressor therapy. Because the pulmonary vasculature constricts when alveolar oxygen tension falls, hypoxemia may provoke decompensation of the right ventricle in patients with cor pulmonale.

Hyperoxia

At normal barometric pressures, venous and tissue oxygen tensions rise very little when pure oxygen is administered to healthy subjects. Hence, non-pulmonary tissues are little affected. However, high concentrations of oxygen eventually replace nitrogen in the lung, even in poorly ventilated regions, causing collapse of low V̇/Q̇ units as oxygen is absorbed by venous blood faster than it is replenished. Diminished lung compliance results. More importantly, high oxygen tensions accelerate the generation of free radicals and other noxious oxidants, injuring bronchial and parenchymal tissue.

The toxic effects of oxygen are both time and concentration dependent. Several hours of pure oxygen breathing are sufficient to cause substernal discomfort due to irritation of bronchial epithelium. In animal experiments, histologic evidence of alveolar injury begins to develop within 12 hours of breathing in an oxygen-rich environment. At high concentrations, parenchymal infiltration and fibrosis eventually occur, a process usually requiring days to weeks. However, there is wide individual variation in susceptibility; many patients undergo no detectable adverse changes under conditions that prove injurious to others. There is general agreement that very high oxygen concentrations are tolerated well for up to 48 hours. At concentrations of inspired oxygen less than 50%, clinically detectable oxygen toxicity is unusual, however long such therapy is required.

CARBON DIOXIDE

Hypercapnia

For the major waste product of oxidative metabolism, CO_2 is a relatively innocuous gas. Apart from its key role in regulation of ventilation, the clinically important effects of CO_2 relate to changes in cerebral blood flow, pH, and adrenergic tone. Hypercapnia dilates cerebral vessels, and hypocapnia constricts them, a point of importance for patients with raised intracranial pressure. Acute increases in CO_2 depress consciousness, probably a result of intraneuronal acidosis. Slowly developing increases in CO_2 are well tolerated, presumably because buffering has time to occur. Nonetheless, a higher $PaCO_2$ signifies alveolar hypoventilation, which tends to cause a decrease in alveolar and arterial PO_2. With hypoxemia and acidosis averted by supplemental oxygen and compensatory alkalosis, some outpatients with $PaCO_2$ levels that chronically exceed 90 mmHg continue to lead active lives. Conversely, patients with renal insufficiency lack the ability to buffer carbonic acid and tolerate hypercapnia poorly.

The adrenergic stimulation that accompanies acute hypercapnia causes cardiac output to rise and peripheral vascular resistance to increase. During acute respiratory acidosis these effects may partially offset those of hydrogen ion on cardiovascular function, allowing better tolerance of low pH than with metabolic acidosis of a similar degree. Constriction of glomerular arterioles also occurs by adrenergic stimulation, producing oliguria in some patients. Muscular twitching, asterixis, and seizures may be observed at extreme levels of hypercapnia in patients made susceptible by electrolyte or neural disorders.

Hypocapnia

The major effects of acute hypocapnia relate to alkalosis and diminished cerebral blood flow. Abrupt lowering of $PaCO_2$ reduces cerebral blood flow and raises neuronal pH, causing altered cortical and peripheral nerve function. Light-headedness, circumoral and fingertip paresthesia, and muscular tetany can result. Sudden major reduction of $PaCO_2$ (e.g., shortly after initiating mechanical ventilation) can produce life-threatening seizures.

HYDROGEN ION CONCENTRATION

For mammalian cells to function optimally, hydrogen ion concentration must be rigidly controlled. The widest range compatible with life is approximately 6.8 - 7.8 pH units.

Acidosis

Although all organs malfunction to some extent during acidosis, cardiovascular function is among the most impaired. Myocardial fibers contract less efficiently, systemic vessels react sluggishly to vasoconstrictive stimuli, vasomotor control deteriorates, blood pressure falls, and arrhythmias develop. (As a result defibrillation and cardiopulmonary resuscitation are especially difficult in an acidotic patient.) In addition, acidosis profoundly impairs neuronal conduction and mental status, acts synergistically with alveolar hypoxia to cause pulmonary vasoconstriction, and blunts the action of adrenergic bronchodilators on the conducting airways. Each of these effects accelerates dramatically in severity as pH falls below 7.20.

Above 7.20, pH is not a major concern in itself and should not prompt therapy aimed solely at pH correction. (In fact, the rightward shift of the oxyhemoglobin curve may improve tissue oxygen delivery if cardiovascular performance remains adequate.) In this higher range, acidosis is more alarming for what it signifies - seriously decompensated ventilatory, metabolic, or cardiovascular systems in need of urgent attention.

Alkalosis

Alkalosis causes less apprehension among physicians than acidosis of a similar degree because the etiology is usually less life-threatening. Raised pH does not exert the dangerously depressing influence on myocardium and blood vessels seen with a similar degree of acidosis. Furthermore, unless very abrupt and severe, the effects of raised pH on the brain are limited to confusion and encephalopathy. The major risk of extreme alkalosis appears to be related to cardiac arrhythmias, which are caused in part by electrolyte shifts (Ca^{++}, K^+) and diminished oxygen delivery. Alkalosis is detrimental with regard to release of oxygen to the tissues, shifting the oxyhemoglobin dissociation curve leftward. As a general rule, pH > 7.60 warrants vigorous measures for reversal.

SUGGESTED READINGS

1. Comroe JH. Physiology of Respiration, 2nd ed. Chicago: Yearbook Medical Publishers, 1974:55-69.

2. Rastegar A, Thier SO. Physiologic consequences and bodily adaptations to hyper and hypocapnea. Chest 1972;62(Suppl):28S-34S.

3. Rose BD. Clinical Physiology of Acid-Base and Electrolyte Disorders, 2nd ed. New York: McGraw-Hill, 1984.

Chapter 5

Acid-Base Physiology

GENERATION AND EXCRETION OF H⁺ ION

To keep H^+ concentration within narrow limits, generation rate must equal elimination rate. H^+ ion is generated in two ways: (1) by hydration of CO_2 to form "volatile" acid according to the reaction:

$$CO_2 + H_2O \rightleftharpoons H_2CO_3 \rightleftharpoons H^+ + HCO_3^-$$

and (2) by production of "fixed" acid (sulfates and phosphates) as a chemical by-product of metabolism. Ventilation eliminates the volatile acid load after reversal of the CO_2 hydration reaction in the lung capillary, while the kidney excretes the bulk of the fixed acid load. If excretion of CO_2 speeds or slows inappropriately, the result is a respiratory derangement of acid-base balance. If the excretion rate of fixed acid speeds or slows disproportionately in relation to production rate, or if abnormal metabolic loads of acid or alkali develop, metabolic acidosis or alkalosis occurs.

BUFFER SYSTEMS

Carbonic Acid

Chemical and protein buffer systems exist in body tissues to oppose changes in free H^+ ion concentration. Of the multiple circulatory buffers, the CO_2/HCO_3^- (carbonic acid) and hemoglobin systems are quantitatively most important. The effect of each buffer pair can be described by an expression equating pH to the ratio of the concentrations of the H^+ acceptor to the H^+ donor. One such equation is the Henderson-Hasselbalch equation:

$$pH = 6.1 + \log (HCO_3^- / .03\ PaCO_2)$$

Clinical attention is focused on the carbonic acid system because each of its components is readily measured and because CO_2 and HCO_3^- determinations allow clinical judgments to be made concerning the respiratory or metabolic origin of the problem at hand. To maintain pH at 7.40, the ratio of HCO_3^- to $(.03 \times PaCO_2)$ must remain at 20:1. Higher or lower ratios indicate high and low pH, respectively.

Protein Buffers

The carbonic acid system does not act in isolation, however. Hemoglobin and other protein buffers also bind or release H^+ ion, minimizing pH changes while allowing the hydration reaction for CO_2 to continue to run in either direction.

$$CO_2 + H_2O \rightleftharpoons H^+ + HCO_3^-$$
$$\quad\quad\quad\quad\quad + Hgb \rightleftharpoons HHb$$

For this reason, if $PaCO_2$ changes acutely, there will be a small associated change in HCO_3^- in the same direction (approximately 1 meq/l per 0.1 pH unit). It is noteworthy that the absence of hemoglobin and other protein buffers in CSF, pleural fluid, urine, and other nonsanguinous body fluids allows pH in them to change dramatically with relatively small changes in H^+ concentration. Anemic blood is a less efficient buffer of fluctuations in H^+ concentration.

Base Excess

Clinically, it is important to be able to quantitate metabolic acid-base derangements. At pH 7.40, simple inspection of the HCO_3^- concentration suffices to detect a metabolic component, whether primary or compensatory for a chronic respiratory disturbance. However, as pH deviates from 7.40, the presence of noncarbonic buffers complicates the interpretation.

The "base excess" is a number that quantitates the metabolic abnormality. It hypothetically "corrects" pH to 7.40 by first "adjusting" $PaCO_2$ to 40 mmHg, thus allowing a comparison of the resultant bicarbonate value with the known normal value at that pH (24 meq/l). As a quick rule of thumb, base excess can be calculated from the observed values for HCO_3^- and pH as:

$$BE_{(meq/l)} = HCO_3^- + 10 (7.40 - pH) - 24$$

A negative base excess means that HCO_3^- stores are depleted. The base excess number does not indicate whether retention or depletion of bicarbonate is pathological or compensatory for long-standing respiratory derangements. That judgment must be made by an analysis of the clinical setting.

COMPENSATORY MECHANISMS

As abnormal stresses on pH balance persist over hours to days, adjustments in the excretion rate of CO_2 and H^+ ion attempt to counterbalance the effect of the disturbance on pH. In general, renal compensation for a respiratory disturbance is slower but ultimately more successful than respiratory compensation for a metabolic disturbance. Thus, although quick to respond, the respiratory system will not eliminate sufficient CO_2 to completely offset any but the mildest metabolic acidosis.

The lower limit of sustained compensatory hypocapnia in a healthy adult appears to be approximately 10-15 mmHg. Once that limit is reached, even small additional increments in H^+ ion have disastrous effects on pH (and survival). Patients with problems of lung mechanics, such as those with COPD and those with neuromuscular weakness, are highly vulnerable to metabolic acid loads because they lack the normal ability to compensate by hyperventilation. CO_2 retention in response to alkalosis is very limited, only rarely exceeding 60 mmHg. The hypoxemia associated with hypoventilation helps limit the rise in CO_2 by triggering increased ventilatory effort.

Although the kidney cannot respond effectively to abrupt respiratory acidosis and alkalosis, renal compensation eventually (3-7 days) may completely counterbalance chronic respiratory alkalosis of moderate severity. The kidney also does relatively well with chronic respiratory acidosis but does not compensate completely for a $PaCO_2$ above 65 mmHg unless another stimulus for HCO_3^- retention is present.

CLASSIFYING ACID-BASE DERANGEMENTS

It is often difficult to be certain whether metabolic causes are primary and respiratory compensation has occurred, or the opposite. The generally valid concept that "compensatory mechanisms never overshoot a normal pH" can be misleading near pH 7.40. For example, acute breath-holding or mild hyperventilation associated with the stress of arterial puncture may cause a pH of 7.42 to drop to 7.38 or the reverse to occur. Mixed alkalosis and acidosis and combined disorders of respiratory and metabolic acidosis (or alkalosis) are frequent problems that must be analyzed using both clinical data and blood gas information. A useful approach is to classify and quantify respiratory and metabolic disturbances and then use clinical observations to identify the likely mechanisms. Using this system, the direction of the respiratory component (respiratory "alkalosis" or "acidosis," respectively) is determined by noting whether $PaCO_2$ is above or below 40 mmHg. Calculating base excess or deficit determines the metabolic component. Clinical judgment then assigns the likely cause for each. For example, in a patient with stable COPD on diuretics, the following values might be obtained: pH = 7.50, $PaCO_2$ = 48 mmHg, HCO_3^- = 36 meq/l, base excess = 11 meq/l. Analysis: mild alkalemia, respiratory acidosis, and metabolic alkalosis. Clinical interpretation: mixed primary disorders of respiratory acidosis and metabolic alkalosis.

SUGGESTED READINGS

1.   Collier CR, Hackney JD, Mohler JG. Use of extracellular base excess in diagnosis of acid-base disorders: a conceptual approach. Chest 1972;61:68-128.

2.   Kassirer JP. Serious acid-base disorders. N. Engl. J. Med. 1974;291:773-76.

3.   Narins RG, et al. Diagnostic strategies in disorders of fluid, electrolyte and acid-base homeostasis. Am. J. Med. 1982;72:496-520.

4.   Rose BD. Clinical Physiology of Acid-Base and Electrolyte Disorders, 2nd ed. McGraw Hill, 1984:202-47.

5.   Woodbury JW. Body acid-base state and its regulation (Chapter 27). In: Ruch TC, Patton HD, eds. Physiology and Biophysics. Circulation, Respiration and Fluid Balance (20th ed.). Philadelphia: Saunders, 1974:480-524.

Chapter 6

Control of Ventilation

The medullary respiratory center modifies its own cyclic rhythm by integrating signals from many sources. These inputs, which may be of cortical, chemical (pH, CO_2, O_2), or reflex origin, cause changes in the timing, frequency, and depth of tidal breathing. In general, each potential modifier of medullary activity is much more potent as a stimulator to increase breathing than as a depressant to retard the endogenous level of ventilation set by the respiratory center. Efferent flow descends via the phrenic nerves to the diaphragm and via the spinal nerves to the intercostal and abdominal muscles.

The precise mechanisms through which the control of ventilation is affected are complex and elusive to define. The background "tone" of the system appears to be set by age, genetic predisposition, and metabolic status. In general, the higher the metabolic rate, the sharper will be the ventilatory response to provocative stimuli (such as hypoxemia or hypercarbia). Starvation suppresses both metabolic rate and drive. Drive improves within hours of refeeding, with protein more effective than carbohydrate or fat in restoring the original set point. Fever and hyperthyroidism intensify central drive, whereas hypothermia and myxedema suppress it.

Control of output from the medullary respiratory center is an interactive process. For example, the precise effect of a given rise in $PaCO_2$ will depend upon the levels of cortical arousal, PaO_2, pH, and mechanoreceptor input. The end result of that neural output will depend upon the ability of the lungs to effect ventilation upon command.

CHEMICAL STIMULI

Medullary H^+ Concentration

Under normal resting conditions, intracerebral hydrogen ion concentration is the predominant influence on ventilatory drive. As in the periphery, the ratio of HCO_3^- concentration to PCO_2 appears to determine pH. Unlike CO_2, which transports passively across the blood-brain barrier, the

HCO_3^- concentration of brain tissue and cerebrospinal fluid is maintained somewhat lower than in blood by an active process (the "brain kidney"). In contrast to its renal counterpart, this mechanism is capable of making relatively rapid compensatory adjustments in HCO_3^- so that CSF pH is restored almost completely to its normal resting value of $\simeq$ 7.32 within 12 hours following derangement. By comparison, CO_2 crosses quickly to the juxtamedullary area. Thus, an abrupt rise in $PaCO_2$ precipitates intracerebral acidosis, prompting increased ventilation to restore pH balance. The potency of an increase in $PaCO_2$ wanes with time, as CSF HCO_3^- rises to compensate. Conversely, the ventilatory compensation for sustained metabolic acidosis is maximized only after 12 or more hours have elapsed following its onset, since peripheral pH receptors initially drive $PaCO_2$ to low levels and create CSF alkalosis that temporarily acts to limit the ventilatory increase.

Hypercarbia

$PaCO_2$ is believed to drive ventilation mainly through its effect on intracerebral H^+ concentration. However, a rise in $PaCO_2$ also stimulates receptors at the carotid bifurcation, perhaps through the peripheral pH receptors located there. The level of PaO_2 modifies the ventilatory response to CO_2, increasing it when hypoxemia occurs. Thus, when hypoxemia is relieved (as during treatment of decompensated COPD), $PaCO_2$ is expected to rise somewhat, even if the respiratory center is otherwise normally responsive to CO_2. The rise in CO_2 will be exaggerated if CO_2 sensitivity is reduced. Cortical depression, whether caused by sleep or sedative drugs, limits the response to CO_2, especially in patients with previously blunted drives.

Prolonged mechanical stress may alter the sensitivity to chemical stimuli. Although the most common example occurs in chronic airflow obstruction, even normal individuals will reset CO_2 drives if made to breathe against resistance for long periods. Teleologically, this occurs because total work of breathing decreases when $PaCO_2$ rises to make each breath more effective.

Hypoxemia

Although an effect can be demonstrated up to 150 mmHg, PaO_2 is an important stimulus for ventilation only when blood is significantly desaturated. Oxygen receptors are located mainly in the carotid body and send signals to the medulla via neural transmission. Extreme hypoxemia blunts rather than stimulates ventilation by direct depression of the medullary center. With advancing age, ventilatory response to hypoxemia and to low blood pH diminishes, perhaps as a consequence of carotid arteriosclerosis. Starvation and sedatives also attenuate hypoxic ventilatory drive.

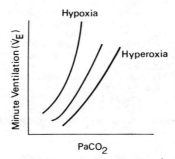

<u>Figure 6.1.</u> Effect of hypercarbia on ventilatory drive (as measured by minute ventilation, $\dot{V}_E$). Hypoxemia exaggerates, and hyperoxemia blunts the normal response.

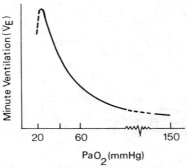

<u>Figure 6.2.</u> Effect of isocapneic hypoxemia on ventilatory drive (as measured by $\dot{V}_E$). Hypoxemia exerts its greatest effect between 25 and 60 mmHg.

<u>Systemic Acidosis</u>

Systemic acidosis is a very potent drive to ventilation, whose effect is at least additive to that of hypoxemia when the two occur together, as they often do clinically. Receptors for peripheral blood pH are located primarily in the carotid body.

NONCHEMICAL STIMULI

Under pathologic stress, neural reflexes originating from receptors located within the lung or chest wall may be the primary driver of ventilation. Thus, the hyperventilation that occurs during the early phases of asthma and pulmonary edema, as well as the chronic hyperventilation of interstitial fibrosis, may result from stimulation of normally quiescent receptors. The importance of thoracic volume to the intensity of these mechanical stimuli is suggested by breath-holding experiments, which demonstrate that apnea endurance declines markedly at low lung volume, independent of chemical inputs. Central neurogenic hyperventilation and Cheyne-Stokes breathing (on average, also a hyperventilatory pattern) result from intracerebral pathology but may be modified by neuromuscular input.

ASSESSING VENTILATORY DRIVE

The sensitivity of the drive center is characterized by its ventilatory response to stimuli. Traditionally, drive assessment has been restricted to hypoxic and hypercapnic stresses applied in the pulmonary function laboratory, using minute ventilation or breathing frequency as the monitored endpoint. Although such methods are valid for patients without lung, chest wall, or muscular impairments, the results are difficult or impossible to interpret when the patient has disordered thoracic mechanics. For example, a patient with obstructive lung disease may retain CO_2 because of a blunted central drive or because of an inability to ventilate, despite powerful neural stimulation. In recent years, increasing use has been made of the pressure generated by the respiratory system very shortly (100 msec) after surreptitious airway occlusion. This $P_{0.1}$ measurement is virtually unaffected by the mechanical characteristics of the chest, because changes in volume do not occur. (Because muscle strength is affected by lung volume, however, FRC must not change markedly between sequential $P_{0.1}$ measurements.) Monitoring of phrenic nerve output is a direct and theoretically appealing approach to assessing central drive, but its implementation is beset with technical problems. At the bedside, only a few measures are practical. Although mean inspiratory flow (V_T/T_i = tidal volume/inspiratory time) is an index of central output in normal subjects, again it is influenced by mechanical and/or neuromuscular impairment. We are left with crude methods to evaluate drive when CO_2 is elevated. What fraction is $\dot{V}_E$ of the patient's ventilatory reserve? Is the patient comfortable or dyspneic? Can $\dot{V}_E$ be dramatically increased by voluntary hyperventilation? Interpretation of these questions against the background of known predisposing factors for drive suppression may allow for a crude but convincing assessment of the intensity of central drive.

CLINICAL DISORDERS OF VENTILATORY CONTROL

For therapeutic purposes, it is important when evaluating hypercapnia to distinguish patients with depressed drives (those who won't breathe) from those whose condition, such as COPD or neuromuscular disease, will not allow them to achieve normal alveolar ventilation (those who can't breathe). Many patients have combined problems of drive and mechanics. For example, because advanced age and starvation may blunt ventilatory drives, an elderly patient with an acutely elevated ventilation requirement and mechanical stress (e.g., pneumonia) often presents with a component of respiratory acidosis as well as hypoxemia. Clues to dysfunction of the primary respiratory center include the absence of obstruction or neuromuscular disease, normal $(A-a)DO_2$, and preserved ability to lower $PaCO_2$ upon command. Because a very wide spectrum of response to $PaCO_2$ and PaO_2 exists even among healthy normal subjects, it is not surprising that two patients with the same pulmonary pathology may set very different levels of alveolar ventilation. Among patients with severe chronic bronchitis there are not only "pink puffers" and "blue bloaters" but also "blue puffers."

Many chronic disorders can depress respiratory center function. Among these, hypothyroidism, malnutrition, and the Pickwickian syndrome are perhaps the most reversible. Responsiveness of central drive to chemical stimuli is restored within hours of refeeding a starved subject. The utility of respiratory center stimulants is limited. Stimulants are contraindicated for patients who retain CO_2 solely because of disordered mechanics or neuromuscular weakness, since dyspnea may worsen with little beneficial effect. Doxapram, a short-acting stimulant of chemoreceptors at both peripheral and central sites, is occasionally useful to avert mechanical ventilation in patients with acute hypoventilation, especially if the precipitating event proves reversible (anesthesia, sedative ingestion). Progesterone increases CO_2 drive in pregnant women and recently has been used therapeutically as a ventilatory stimulant for primary hypoventilation. Its maximal effect is delayed several days after beginning treatment.

SUGGESTED READINGS

1. Berger AS, Mitchell RA, Severinghouse JW. Regulation of respiration (Three parts). N. Engl. J. Med. 1977;297:92-97, 138-143, 194-201.

2.   Fishman AP, Cherniack NS, Widdicombe JG, eds. Control of Breathing (Volume 2 of the Respiratory System, Section 3). In: Handbook of Physiology. Bethesda: American Physiological Society, 1986.

3.   Hornbein TF, ed. Regulation of Breathing (Volume 17 In: Lung Biology in Health and Disease Series). New York: Marcel Dekker, 1982.

4.   Whitelaw WA, Derenne JP, Milic-Emili J. Occlusion pressure as a measure of respiratory center output in conscious man. Respir. Physiol. 1975;23:181-99.

5.   Williams MH, ed. Disturbance of respiratory control (symposium). Clin. Chest Med. 1980;1:1-159.

6.   Wyman RJ. Neural generation of the breathing rhythm. Ann. Rev. Physiol. 1977;39:417-48.

Chapter 7

Physical Examination

SYMPTOMS

Dyspnea

Dyspnea is a subjective complaint that arises when disproportionate effort is felt to be necessary to achieve adequate ventilation. It is a complex sensation mediated by a variety of disparate parenchymal, vascular, neuro-muscular, and supratentorial inputs. Yet, one unifying and commonly held theory suggests that dyspnea usually results when the force applied to the chest by the respiratory muscles does not produce sufficient volume change to satisfy mechanoreceptors embedded in the lung and/or chest wall. The interrelationship between the changes in muscle fiber length and tension appears to be the key. For example, the respiratory muscles can work very hard during exercise without provoking unpleasant sensations because changes in length and tension remain appropriate.

Because of the normally wide margin between resting ventilatory requirement and maximal breathing capacity, exertional dyspnea is usually the earliest manifestation of diminished reserves. Disproportionate exercise dyspnea is particularly characteristic of upper airway obstruction, exercise-induced asthma, and advanced pulmonary hypertension. Nocturnal dyspnea characterizes asthma, COPD, and congestive heart failure (CHF).

Chest Pain

Pleurisy, a product of infectious, neoplastic, or embolic events, is not the only type of lung-related chest pain. Although lung parenchyma and visceral pleura are not invested with pain fibers, a dull, continuous substernal ache is experienced during acute irritation of the central airways, as during bronchitis or exercise in cold air. A similar sensation may be felt during acute exacerbations of pulmonary hypertension, occasionally causing confusion with myocardial infarction or exertional angina. Mediastinal and peribronchial disease (e.g., due to lung cancer) can cause deep central or unilateral pain.

Herpes zoster of intercostal nerve roots often presents first with segmental pain and/or tenderness, even before skin lesions are evident. Vigorous coughing often culminates in painful spasm or injury of intercostal or diaphragmatic muscle fibers. Stress fractures of the ribs, undetectable by routine chest films, can also occur.

Orthopnea

Left heart failure is the best known cause of orthopnea but not the only one:

Hypoxemia often worsens while recumbent, especially in obese patients with diseased airways. Desaturation occurs as resting lung volume (FRC) falls, allowing a portion of each tidal breath to occur with some airways closed to ventilation. (FRC exceeds closing volume.)

Decreased lung volume when supine may cause airways to narrow sufficiently to produce dyspnea related to obstruction or air trapping.

Pulmonary hypertension may worsen as the increased blood flow or hypoxemia of the supine position boosts pressures in a restricted pulmonary vascular bed.

Recumbency dramatically impairs ventilatory function in patients with diaphragmatic paralysis or massive obesity.

In contrast, some patients may experience dyspnea upon assuming an upright position. Usually the explanation is neuromuscular in origin. Rarely, however, desaturation of arterial blood occurs (orthodeoxia). This phenomenon has been described in patients with cirrhosis, arteriovenous malformations, and in the postpneumonectomy period. Its explanation remains obscure but likely relates to gravitational rerouting of mixed venous blood to poorly ventilated basilar units or in some cases through abnormal basilar vascular malformations or intracardiac shunt pathways.

Cough (See Chapter 25)

Causes

Stimulation of irritant receptors in the nasopharynx, larynx, and lower airway can trigger involuntary cough. Among the most common causes of persistent unexplained coughing are postviral, allergic, or chronic bronchitis, asthma, sinusitis, smoking, postnasal drip, esophageal reflux with or without aspiration, swallowing dysfunction, tuberculosis, and endobronchial tumors.

Diagnostic Clues

Postnasal drip may be unaccompanied by tussive symptoms during the day, only to emerge as a major problem shortly after assuming recumbency. Cough may be deeply productive upon rising. A productive cough, worse in the morning, suggests chronic bronchitis. Except during infective or allergic exacerbations, the sputum is not purulent. Copious unrelenting production of purulent phlegm suggests bronchiectasis or lung abscess. Hoarseness in association with cough suggests vocal cord compression or inflammation. Chronic nocturnal aspiration of oropharyngeal secretions or gastric material may be a subtle and vexing problem - always ask about reflux symptoms. "Brassy" cough suggests major airway compression, whereas a "bovine" cough suggests vocal cord paralysis. Allergic bronchitis is a surprisingly common and underdiagnosed condition, even in the absence of asthmatic symptoms. Examination of the retropharynx, nasal turbinates, nasal secretions, and expectorated sputum for eosinophils may provide essential clues. Coughing during meals suggests aspiration, either due to swallowing dysfunction or (rarely) tracheoesophageal communication. Coughing during sleep suggests aspiration of pooled oral secretions or gastric contents. Exercise-induced coughing can represent an asthma or anginal equivalent. Positional variation may characterize a cough of cardiac origin.

PHYSICAL FINDINGS - Pulmonary

Breathing Pattern

The ventilation accomplished per minute ($\dot{V}_E$) is the product of tidal volume (V_t) and frequency (f): $\dot{V}_E = V_t \times f$. Since f can be expressed as the reciprocal of cycle length (T_{tot}), this equation can be expressed $\dot{V}_E = V_t/T_i \times T_i/T_{tot}$, where T_i is the inspiratory time. V_t/T_i, the mean inspiratory flow rate, is a useful measure of respiratory drive in patients without mechanical impairment. T_i/T_{tot}, variably known as the inspiratory cycle length, duty cycle, or fractional inspiratory time, varies with disease type and level of ventilation.

Normally, $V_t/T_i \simeq 15$ liters/min, $T_i/T_{tot} \simeq 0.4$, and $f \simeq 16$/min. Restrictive lung disease usually elevates drive (V_t/T_i) and respiratory rate, but values for V_t and T_i/T_{tot} remain within the normal range. In moderate to severe obstruction, f, V_t, and V_t/T_i each increase and T_i/T_{tot} falls. Normally, the rib cage and abdominal compartments move in varying proportions, depending on position, body habitus, and level of ventilatory stress. During quiet inspiration in the supine position, outward abdominal motion predominates. As breathing becomes vigorous, however, inspiratory rib cage excursions over-balance abdominal movements, and under severe stress, the abdomen may even move inward paradoxically. Paradoxical motion of the abdominal wall in the recumbent position during quiet breathing is a cardinal sign of bilateral diaphragmatic paralysis. Asynchronous excursions of the thorax and abdomen characterize many patients with COPD and those on the threshold of respiratory muscle exhaustion.

Symmetrical inward motion of the lower ribs at the start of inhalation is occasionally seen in patients with severe airflow obstruction as the fibers of the flattened diaphragm contract to pull their attachments centrally (Hoover's sign). Intercostal retractions and active use of the accessory muscles of ventilation signify a major ventilatory work load. Contraction of the expiratory muscles is required at high ventilatory levels and when breathing against high resistive loads. Palpation of the upper abdomen can detect active tension of the powerful rectus group. Paradoxical motion of the sternum or segments of the thoracic cage during inhalation usually indicates a region broken free from its attachments by traumatic injury.

Breath Sounds

Auscultation is performed by comparing each region with that of the opposite lung, not by moving top to bottom. The patient should be instructed to breathe deeply through an open mouth. Diminished or absent (but not normal quality) breath sounds are consistent with severe airflow obstruction.

Basilar rales (crackles) that disappear after several deep breaths denote microatelectasis. Auscultation should start at the bases during quiet breathing in order to detect these rales before deep tidal excursions obliterate them.

Crackles of COPD usually begin early in inspiration and continue throughout. Basilar crackles that begin late in inspiration ("Velcro" rales) are most consistent with interstitial fibrosis.

Consolidation diminishes breath sounds only if secretions block conducting airways. "Tubular" (or bronchial) breathing indicates patency of the bronchus.

Egophony (E to A changes) may be heard over partially aerated but compressed tissue, most frequently above a pleural effusion.

Secretions in conducting airways produce rhonchi. Although usually inspiratory, rhonchi may be heard throughout the cycle when secretions fill large airways. Occasionally, differentiation of a rhonchus from a pleural rub may prove difficult. Rhonchi tend to clear with coughing and are heard mainly in inspiration, whereas rubs are more localized, usually associated with pain, and heard during both phases of the ventilatory cycle.

Wheezes

Wheezing is a musical high-pitched sound caused by rapid airflow through critically narrowed airways, ordinarily arising as airways are compressed during exhalation. Unilateral wheezing and wheezing heard throughout the ventilatory cycle suggest fixed bronchial narrowing.

Apart from asthma, wheezes accompany COPD, left heart congestive failure, pulmonary embolism, upper airway obstruction, and bronchogenic carcinoma.

Wheezes are often best heard with the patient recumbent, since reduced lung volume may cause the requisite critical narrowing to occur.

The absence of wheezing during deep but unforced breathing in patients with chronic airflow obstruction usually means little responsiveness to inhaled bronchodilators. Although very loud wheezing usually indicates a large reversible component, wheezing can be heard with irreversible obstruction as well.

Mild wheezing heard during forced exhalation is common among patients without obstructive lung disease, limiting the diagnostic value of this maneuver. On the contrary, the absence of forced wheezing is very uncommon in obstructive lung disease and suggests either submaximal effort or severe emphysema.

Forced Expiratory Time (FET)

With normal rates of airflow, a stethoscope placed over the trachea will detect audible airflow for three seconds or less after the start of a forced vital capacity maneuver. If sound persists longer than six seconds, at least moderate obstruction is present.

Stridor

Variable extrathoracic and fixed upper airway obstructions cause stridor, a prolonged, shrill, crowing noise heard during inspiration. The intensity of stridor is dependent on the forcefulness of the inspiratory effort. Upper airway obstruction may complicate asthma or masquerade as asthma refractory to bronchodilator therapy. The detection of true stridor should prompt a careful but expeditious evaluation of the upper airway, since obstruction must generally be severe to produce this sign. Secretions pooled in the retropharynx can produce loud inspiratory sounds that mimic stridor, without the same ominous significance.

Percussion

Asymmetrical dullness to percussion can result from underlying fluid, consolidation, atelectasis, or displacement of the abdominal contents into the chest. Failure of the uppermost margin of dullness to change with deep inspiration suggests diaphragmatic immobility. Auscultation and re-percussion in the lateral decubitus position are useful methods of differentiating among these alternative diagnoses when the chest film leaves room for doubt. Unilateral hyperresonance is suggestive of pneumothorax or, conversely, infiltration of the contralateral lung or pleural space.

PHYSICAL FINDINGS - Extrapulmonary

Careful examination of the heart, neck veins, and lower extremities is important in separating cardiovascular from pulmonary disease. Cyanosis results from an increased concentration of reduced hemoglobin circulating in dermal venules. Therefore, it may result from inadequate arterial oxygenation or increased capillary extraction of oxygen, whatever the etiology. Impaired pulmonary gas exchange and circulatory stagnation (due to vasoconstriction or reduced cardiac output) are the primary causes. Methemoglobinemia is an unusual cause for cyanosis unrelated to either of these mechanisms. Drug ingestion in predisposed persons may reduce oxygen-carrying capacity by oxidizing ferrous iron within the hemoglobin molecule.

Frequently neglected portions of the physical examination bear special relevance to pulmonary complaints. Examination of the nasal passages, tympanic membranes, and sinuses may disclose a source for the mucous drainage that provokes asthma or chronic cough. A depressed gag reflex may indicate a predisposition to chronic aspiration of ingested food or oral secretions. In the setting of hoarseness or a recent voice change, indirect laryngoscopy frequently reveals cord paralysis or inflammation, findings compatible with intrathoracic neoplasia or reflux/aspiration, respectively. Telangiectasis of the nasal, conjunctival, or mucous membranes may provide clues to the presence of pulmonary arteriovenous communications or to the origin of unexplained hemoptysis. Whenever thoracic neoplasia is suspected, the supraclavicular fossae should be probed with special care, using a Valsalva maneuver when necessary to elevate the nodes toward the clavicular level. Inspection and palpation of the fingers, toes, wrists, and long bones can reveal the swelling and tenderness characteristic of hypertrophic osteoarthropathy or collagen vascular disease. Localized chest wall tenderness may reflect nerve root or muscular inflammation or an underlying rib fracture. The latter is particularly likely if sternospinal compression generates intense pain laterally, remote from the direct site of pressure.

SUGGESTED READINGS

1. Altose MD. Dyspnea (Chapter 7). In: Simmons DH, ed. Current Pulmonology (Volume 7). Chicago: Yearbook Medical Publishers, 1986:199-226.

2. Christopher KL, et al. Vocal cord dysfunction presenting as asthma. N. Engl. J. Med. 1983;308:1566-70.

3. Fishman AP. Manifestations of respiratory disorders (Chapter 3). In: Fishman AP, ed. Pulmonary Diseases and Disorders. New York: McGraw-Hill, 1980:44-83.

4. Forgacs P. The functional basis of pulmonary sounds. Chest 1978;73:399-405.

5. Irwin RS, Rosen, MJ, Braman SS. Cough a comprehensive review. Arch. Int. Med. 1977;137:1186-91.

6. Marini JJ, Pierson DJ, Hudson LD, et al. The significance of wheezing in chronic airflow obstruction. Am. Rev. Respir. Dis. 1979;120:1069-72.

7. McFadden ER. Acute bronchial asthma. Relations between clinical and physiologic manifestations. N. Engl. J. Med. 1973;288:221-25.

Chapter 8

Blood Gas Sampling and Noninvasive Measurement

METHODS FOR ASSESSING PaO$_2$

Analysis of arterial and mixed venous blood can provide vital information concerning respiratory, cardiac, and metabolic function. Although arterial blood has a uniform composition, venous samples from various organs differ widely in their content of O$_2$ and CO$_2$. Furthermore, the perfusion, metabolic status, and venous O$_2$ content of any individual organ can fluctuate markedly over time. Thus, for calculations of overall oxygen consumption or extraction, venous blood must be withdrawn from the pulmonary artery after all samples have been mixed by the right ventricle.

Alternatives to Arterial Puncture

Noninvasive oximetry with a pulse or earlobe sensor enables continuous noninvasive estimation of arterial oxygen saturation. This proves useful during anesthesia and bronchoscopy, as well as during studies of sleep and exercise. In the critical care setting, oximetry permits rapid evaluation of the response to administered oxygen, to changes in ventilator settings, and to PEEP application. Extreme jaundice (bilirubin > 15 mg/dl) and low cardiac output may cause underestimation of true arterial saturation. Oximetry is insensitive to changes in oxygen tension for saturations at both extremes of the PaO$_2$ range.

Transcutaneous oxygen monitoring is a useful modality for infants but cannot be confidently applied to the adult population. For optimal performance this technique demands luxuriant, homogenous perfusion and high dermal permeability, characteristics lacking in the adult skin. Transcutaneous CO$_2$ monitoring shares many of these same characteristics. Although neither can be considered entirely suitable for arterial gas monitoring in adult patients, both may eventually prove useful as sensors of global perfusion adequacy in critical illness and to monitor local ischemia in surgical applications.

COMPLICATIONS OF INVASIVE SAMPLING

Complications of Puncture

Significant local bleeding should not occur if firm pressure is applied for sufficient time over the puncture site. Adequate time of compression can only be judged by inspecting the site after pressure release. Patients should not be asked to perform these assessments.

Because the hand is normally perfused by two interconnecting arteries, ischemic consequences of radial puncture are rare, especially when patency of the ulnar artery is confirmed, a small-gauge needle is used, and the same site is not punctured repeatedly. Brachial and femoral artery punctures carry a higher risk for ischemic (thrombotic or embolic) consequences and for occult bleeding. Inexpert attempts to puncture the artery may cause nerve trauma at any site.

Complications of Cannulation

Risks of bleeding, thrombosis, and digital ischemia are higher for arterial cannulation than for puncture. Wrist circumference correlates directly with the size of the radial artery lumen and hence inversely with the likelihood of thrombosis. Although the cumulative risk of thrombosis increases rapidly with the duration of cannulation during the first 24 hours, it rises more slowly thereafter. Femoral arterial lines are preferred by many physicians for their improved accuracy in reflecting central pressures.

Indwelling arterial cannulae are either sealed with a stopcock and filled with heparinized saline (heparin lock) or connected to an arterial pressure transducer and high-pressure infusion set. All connections must be taped securely to avoid disassembly and massive bleeding. Frequent, direct observation of the patient is essential whenever an arterial line is in place. Rhythm and blood pressure monitoring are highly desirable to avoid serious consequences if hemorrhage should occur.

Vigorous flushing of radial catheters has been reported to cause cerebral embolization of clots. This may happen because radial and aortic root pressures are similar. Gentle irrigation with small (2-ml or less) boluses of liquid will obviate this problem.

Localized infection becomes increasingly likely after 72 hours of cannulation. Assiduous wound and dressing care and the earliest possible removal of the catheter minimize the risk.

POINTS OF TECHNIQUE: SAMPLING

Without altering F_iO_2, place the patient in the desired position for 10-20 minutes before the sample is drawn (depending on the severity of underlying lung disease). Shorter times may not allow steady-state conditions to be achieved. It is particularly important to note the position of the patient, because positional changes in venous admixture can cause notable differences among serial values of PaO_2.

Arterial Puncture

The preferred site for puncture is the radial artery, but the brachial and femoral arteries can also be used with an escalating risk of nerve trauma and occult bleeding. Although the risk of thrombosis in these larger arteries is less, the potential consequences of occlusion are more severe.

Approximately 3% of hospitalized patients have inadequate collateral flow to the hand. Perform an Allen test for collateral flow by asking the patient to make a fist while both radial and ulnar arteries are tightly occluded by digital pressure. When the open hand blanches white, release only the ulnar compression. The color should flush to normal within 5-7 seconds. If it does not, inadequate collateral circulation may permit serious ischemia during radial vessel spasm or thrombosis. Doppler examination and finger plethysmography are excellent alternatives in hospitals equipped with such devices.

The radial site is swabbed first with povidone-iodine solution, then wiped once with alcohol. A skin wheal of 1% lidocaine is raised over the pulsatile radial artery with a 25-gauge needle. The inner surface of the 3-ml sampling syringe is coated with heparin (1000 units/ml) by drawing up 0.5 ml and then rotating and working the plunger the full length of the barrel several times. Since the dead space of a 21-gauge needle and 3-ml syringe is approximately 0.15 ml, an adequate amount of heparin remains to anticoagulate a 2-ml specimen after the syringe has been emptied.

The patient should be reassured and advised to breathe as normally as possible. With the syringe held at a 45° angle over the dorsiflexed wrist, the radial artery is located with gentle, nonocclusive pressure from the forefinger of the opposite hand. The skin is pierced at the wheal site, and the needle tip enters the artery at a point just distal to the palpating finger. When entry is signaled by the spontaneous appearance of blood in the syringe, the needle is held steady until 1-2 ml of blood are obtained. Let the syringe fill by itself - do not aspirate. Occasionally the needle tip will leave the lumen, most often because downward pressure has caused the needle to penetrate the dorsal arterial wall. Withdrawing the needle very slowly usually re-establishes flow. After sampling, withdraw the needle from the wrist as the radial artery is occluded by the palpating forefinger. Maintain firm pressure at least 5 minutes (longer if the patient has any clotting abnormality). Express any air bubbles from the syringe, cork it, and roll the barrel between the fingers to thoroughly mix the blood with heparin. (Removing the needle and capping the hub is an alternative to corking.) Ice the sample, recording time, position, F_iO_2, and identifying data, and deliver it quickly to the laboratory.

Puncture at brachial and femoral sites is similar, but the angle of entry steepens to 60° and 75°, respectively. It is best to plot the course of the brachial artery segment by using the separated index and second fingers to determine its line before puncture is attempted. Following puncture, the arm should not be bent when applying pressure.

Arterial Cannulation

Cannulation facilitates management when continuous blood pressure monitoring or multiple arterial blood gas determinations are needed. Quick and relatively atraumatic, percutaneous entry using an 18- or 20-gauge plastic cannula over an internal needle guide is preferable to cutdown technique. The smaller catheter is preferred for its dynamic response characteristics and lower risk of thrombosis. The wrist is dorsiflexed over a towel pad, and the palm and upper forearm are taped loosely to an arm board. Lidocaine (1-2 ml of 2%) is used to raise a small skin wheal and to infiltrate the area after the radial site has been prepared with povidone-iodine and alcohol scrubs. (Infiltration with lidocaine helps to avoid arterial spasm during placement.) A 10-ml syringe is prepared, tipped with a stopcock, and filled with 3-5 ml of heparinized saline (50 units per ml).

Just as for arterial puncture, the skin is pierced at a 45° angle and the artery is entered. Using the transfixation method, the needle is advanced to puncture the far wall of the artery and then removed, leaving the cannula in place. The cannula is then slowly withdrawn until blood spurts freely from the open end. Next, the cannula is advanced up the artery and the syringe is used to flush the cannula slowly with 2 ml of solution. The stopcock is turned to seal the artery, and the syringe is removed. Connections are made to the transducer and high-pressure infusion set. Finally, the cannula and all connections are taped, the pad removed, and the armboard secured.

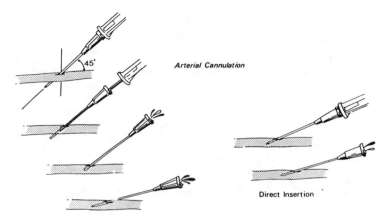

Figure 8.1. Arterial cannulation: two methods.

The artery can also be entered directly using a shallower angle of insertion. However, the needle tip must be advanced well into the artery so that the cannula remains within the lumen as the needle is withdrawn. A newer method employs a modified Seldinger technique. After the artery is entered, a guidewire is passed into the artery. The plastic cannula is then advanced into position over the guidewire.

POINTS OF TECHNIQUE: MEASUREMENT

Delayed Analysis

Samples must be submitted for analysis soon after they are drawn. In a capped but un-iced sample, $PaCO_2$ rises by 3-10 mmHg/hour and pH falls modestly because of ongoing cellular metabolism. (The rates of change depend on the leukocyte count.) Simultaneously, PaO_2 falls by an amount that varies directly with the initial value. An iced sample retains its initial tensions acceptably well for 1-2 hours. Body fluids other than blood are depleted of protein and hemoglobin buffers, so that the pH of an un-iced sample may fall dramatically over a short time.

Excessive Heparin

At normal arterial oxygen tensions, either glass or plastic syringes may be used. At high arterial oxygen tensions, plastic syringes are significantly permeable to oxygen, and glass is preferred. Although heparin is mildly acidic (pH approximately 7.0), the major effect of heparin is dilutional. Large amounts of heparin tend to decrease the HCO_3^- and $PaCO_2$ of the sample almost in proportion to one another, so that pH usually remains unchanged.

Air Bubbles

At sea level, room air has a PO_2 and PCO_2 of 150 and 0 mmHg. Hence, if an air bubble is large and well mixed with the sample, $PaCO_2$ falls very slightly, and PaO_2 will rise 0-30 mmHg in direct relationship to the original PaO_2 and hemoglobin concentration relative to bubble size. However, bubbles are usually of little consequence if quickly expelled because their O_2 does not rapidly equilibrate with the blood sample and their volume is relatively small.

Fever and Hypothermia

Analyzed at the machine temperature of 37°C, blood samples uncorrected for temperature will have gas tensions that differ from those actually present in a febrile or hypothermic patient. This occurs because warming shifts the oxyhemoglobin dissociation curve rightward, whereas cooling causes a leftward shift. Thus, for the same oxygen content, PO_2 will be higher in a warm environment than a cold one. PCO_2 will also be higher when the sample is warm because a higher tension is required to keep CO_2 in solution. (The pH will consequently fall slightly.) Except during severe hypothermia, these corrections are relatively small, and many good laboratories do not correct routinely for temperature.

Hyperventilation and Breath-holding

Occasionally, the blood gas values obtained from anxious patients who hyperventilate or arrest breathing during a difficult arterial puncture can lead to erroneous clinical impressions. For example, a breath-holding patient with weak hypoxic ventilatory drive may allow PaO_2 to fall to an alarming value during apnea. Although some care must be taken during sampling to avoid disruption of the normal breathing pattern and to take note of obvious departures, minor aberrations are usually inconsequential to the analysis.

SUGGESTED READINGS

1. Kelman GR, Nunn JF. Nomograms for correction of blood PO_2, PCO_2, pH, and base excess for time and temperature. J. Appl. Physiol. 1966;21:1484-90.

2. Mueller RG, Long GE, Beam JM. Bubbles in samples for blood gas determinations. Am. J. Clin. Pathol. 1976;65:242-49.

3. Shapiro BA, Harrison RA, Walton JR. Clinical Application of Blood Gases, 3rd ed. Yearbook Medical Publishers, Chicago, 1982.

4. Tremper KK, Shoemaker WC. Transcutaneous oxygen monitoring of critically-ill adults with and without low-flow shock. Crit. Care Med. 1981;9:706-09.

5. Wiedemann HP, Matthay MA, Matthay RA. Cardiovascular pulmonary monitoring in the intensive care unit. Chest 1984;85:537-49.

Chapter 9

Thoracentesis

INDICATIONS

Most undiagnosed fluid collections large enough to be demonstrated easily on an upright chest x-ray (indicating a minimum of 200 ml) should be sampled for diagnostic purposes, especially if the potential for infection exists. In patients with underlying lung or heart disease, removal of modest quantities of pleural fluid can temporarily relieve dyspnea (therapeutic thoracentesis) while other more definitive therapy is begun.

COMPLICATIONS

Pneumothorax

Air may enter through the needle at the time of the procedure, especially when an attempt is made to withdraw a large amount of fluid (therapeutic thoracentesis). The volume of air is usually small and will be reabsorbed spontaneously.

Laceration of the visceral pleura is a more serious problem and usually occurs toward the end of the procedure as the expanding lung approaches the chest wall. Use of a flexible catheter nearly obviates this risk.

Bilateral effusions should not be tapped at the same sitting without an intervening chest film to document the result of the first procedure.

Hypoxemia

As compressed lung distends, perfusion to this newly expanded area improves while ventilation remains inhomogenous. The result is $\dot{V}/\dot{Q}$ mismatch and hypoxemia.

Vasovagal Reflex

Uncommonly, hypotension, bradycardia, nausea, and vomiting may occur. Atropine sulfate (0.8 mg IM) given 10 minutes before the procedure minimizes this risk. Peripheral vasodilation and hypotension, unaccompanied by bradycardia or other stigmata of vagal stimulation, may also occur and often do not respond to anticholinergic therapy (atropine). Maintaining the patient in a horizontal posture is prudent until vasoparesis reverses.

Re-expansion Pulmonary Edema

Rapid removal of large amounts of fluid from a patient with a long-standing effusion can cause hydrostatic edema of the expanded lung. Limiting the volume withdrawn at a single time to 1000 ml and using gentle suction appear to prevent the clinical syndrome. Because pulmonary edema rarely occurs following insertion of a chest tube or drainage of large quantities of fluid by gentle suction, pulling very negative pressure at the time of thoracentesis (usually at the end of the procedure) appears to be a causative factor in some cases.

Intra-abdominal Injury

Low needle placement may cause laceration of liver or spleen, with potentially disastrous consequences. The needle should not be inserted below the 7th, 8th, or 10th ribs in the anterior midclavicular, midaxillary, or posterior scapular lines, respectively. The needle should be directed slightly cephalad. Liver puncture is usually better tolerated than spleen puncture.

Neural Injury and Hemothorax

Adherence to proper needle placement (avoiding the underside of the rib) will obviate this risk. Patients with a bleeding diathesis should not undergo thoracentesis until the hemostatic defect has been corrected.

Bacterial Contamination of Pleural Fluid

This occurs very rarely with good site preparation and aseptic technique. Nonetheless, the site of puncture must not be infected (pyoderma, herpes zoster). In theory, needle puncture of an underlying infected lung may introduce a large innoculum and precipitate empyema. This risk is minimized by appropriate antibiotic coverage and by limiting the diagnostic tap of a parapneumonic effusion to small (50 ml) samples. Thoracentesis should be avoided postpneumonectomy unless empyema is strongly suspected.

Needle Tract Seeding by Tumor Cells

Thoracentesis almost never precipitates this problem. When it does occur, mesothelioma is the usual setting.

POINTS OF TECHNIQUE

Verify that fluid is accessible to the needle with a lateral decubitus film or, if a supine CT is already available, look for a fluid layer posteriorly. Verification is especially important when subdiaphragmatic fluid is suspected.

If a density is immobile and presumed to be loculated fluid, ultrasonography or computed tomography of the pleural space will confirm its nature and map the appropriate region for a pleural tap.

Fluoroscopy at the time of the procedure may be used to guide the needle if the effusion is small and difficult to enter.

Supplemental oxygen should be provided if a large amount of fluid is to be removed.

By the posterior approach, identify the highest interspace of dullness at the end of a normal (not deep) inspiration and (after sterile site preparation) enter just over the top of the lower rib defining this interspace just medial to the posterior axillary line.

Anteriorly, use the midclavicular line, entering the midportion of the interspace to avoid vessels and nerves.

Adequate local anesthesia is mandatory and is achieved by carefully anesthetizing the rib periosteum and parietal pleura with 5-15 ml of 2% lidocaine, using a 22-gauge needle. Advance cautiously, 1-2 mm at a time, avoiding intravascular injection by periodically attempting to aspirate blood beforehand. Confirm the presence of fluid and adequate anesthesia by entering the pleural space and withdrawing fluid at the end of anesthesia.

Thoracentesis of ordinary fluids can usually be done through a 1½-inch long 20-gauge needle. Although the great majority of fluids can be sampled with needles of this length and caliber, very thick fluids may require 18- or even 16-gauge needles to allow easy aspiration and continued patency. Very long (spinal) needles may be required if the skin and subcutaneous tissues are unusually generous or if a thick pleural rind separates the ribs from the liquid pocket. If the intention is to drain the pleural space completely (of either air or fluid), this is better achieved with a thin, <u>flexible</u> <u>catheter</u>. The disadvantage of these catheters, however, is that they kink easily and often obstruct prematurely, closed with fibrin. Because of their innately high resistance, they are less likely to transmit sustained, highly negative pressures to the pleural space until the very end of the procedure. Needles with external plastic sheaths also work well but often kink.

<u>Gentle</u> <u>suction</u> recovers fluid more easily (and safely) than strong suction, which may cause the needle to clog with tissue and possibly precipitate re-expansion edema. For these reasons the use of plasma collection bottles with wide-bore needles and collapse-resistant tubing should be discouraged.

A "<u>dry</u> <u>tap</u>" when a large effusion is clearly present on x-ray usually means one of the following:

Cause	Remedy
a thick pleural rind or chest wall	use a longer needle
loculation	probe a different area, under guidance if necessary
improper needle placement	choose a different interspace
blocked needle	withdraw needle, clear lumen, or replace

<u>Heparinize</u> the <u>container</u> into which fluid is collected (1000 u/liter). Otherwise, cell and protein determinations may be compromised by clotting of proteinaceous fluids.

<u>Coughing</u> after several hundred ml have been recovered usually signifies irritation of re-expanded terminal airways or a pneumothorax. Persistent coughing enhances the risk of pneumothorax and should prompt needle removal.

Thirty to 50 ml should be removed for routine diagnosis (chemistry, hematology, cytology, bacteriology), up to 300 ml for optimal cytologic yield, and 500-1500 ml for relief of dyspnea or TB culture. Specimens should be processed rapidly.

In an asymptomatic patient, a postprocedure film may not be needed after a brief and uncomplicated diagnostic procedure. After a therapeutic tap, however, a <u>postprocedure film</u> should be obtained to establish the new baseline condition. However, filming should be delayed by 1-2 hours to allow a lung-puncture pneumothorax or re-expansion edema to manifest, unless the patient exhibits symptoms beforehand.

An obviously <u>bloody fluid</u> that does not clear as the tap proceeds should prompt immediate (as the procedure continues) analysis for xanthochromia and erythrocyte crenation - signs of a preexisting bloody effusion. Lack of these findings strongly suggests vessel or organ entry.

<u>Routine diagnostic tests</u> are glucose, protein, cell count and differential, and LDH (see p. 209). Bacterial culture, cytology, and complement determinations require special preparation and handling. When clinically indicated, pH determination requires direct withdrawal of the specimen from the pleural space, immediate icing, and rapid analysis.

A <u>simultaneous blood sample</u> should be analyzed for protein, LDH, and glucose.

SUGGESTED READINGS

1.   Leff A, Hopewell PD, Costello J. Pleural effusion from malignancy. <u>Ann. Int. Med.</u> 1978;88:532-37.

2.   Light RW. <u>Pleural Diseases</u>. Philadelphia: Lea and Febiger, 1983.

3.   Light RW, et al. The diagnostic separation of transudates and exudates. <u>Ann. Int. Med.</u> 1972;77:507-13.

4.   Light RW, et al. Observations on pleural fluid pressures as fluid is withdrawn during thoracentesis. <u>Am. Rev. Respir. Dis.</u> 1980;121:799-804.

5.   Pavlin DJ. Lung re-expansion - for better or worse? <u>Chest</u> 1986;89:2-3.

Pleural Biopsy

INDICATIONS

Biopsy of the parietal pleura can establish a diagnosis of pleural tuberculosis or malignancy. In both conditions, obtaining pleural tissue improves the diagnostic yield of fluid analysis by 50-100%. Nonetheless, approximately one-third of pleural fluids caused by malignancy and one-quarter of those caused by tuberculosis remain undiagnosed after complete analysis (and culture) of both fluid and closed parietal biopsy. A partial explanation is that malignancy may cause pleural fluid by congestion of mediastinal lymphatics, by infection, or by selective involvement of the visceral pleura, as well as by invading the parietal pleura. In addition, both tuberculosis and malignancy commonly involve the pleura in a patchy fashion, so that whether an infiltrated area is recovered on closed biopsy depends a bit on luck. (Open biopsy and thoracoscopy are two ways to improve the yield.)

If the first set of three-quadrant biopsies are nondiagnostic, a second procedure will establish the diagnosis approximately 25% of the time, provided that pleural tissue is obtained on both occasions. Further attempts beyond two are usually unrewarding. Often the exact histologic type of tumor cannot be determined with certainty from the small bits of tissue obtained. This is especially true of mesothelioma, in which case even open pleural biopsy may not establish the histologic diagnosis with certainty.

COMPLICATIONS

Although all of the complications listed for thoracentesis may occur and are somewhat more frequent, pneumothorax deserves special mention because manipulation of the needle components is particularly likely to introduce air. An unintentional lung biopsy is all too easily obtained by hooking or aspirating parenchyma.

Attempts at pleural biopsy are contraindicated in the absence of either sufficient fluid to separate the pleural layers or thickened pleura densely adherent to the chest wall. Biopsy should definitely not be attempted in patients with an uncorrected coagulation problem.

Biopsy of neurovascular bundle elements can cause major hemothorax or neural injury.

Repeated attempts can macerate skin and subcutaneous tissues sufficiently to encourage infection. Careful technique and gentle approximation of the incision with sterile tape (Steri-Strips) and nonocclusive dressing will minimize the risk.

POINTS OF TECHNIQUE

Atropine (0.8-1.2 mg IM) helps to counteract the vagal stimulation that can cause bradycardia, hypotension, nausea, or vomiting.

Without direct supervision, pleural biopsy should not be attempted by personnel who are not thoroughly experienced with the use of the available instrument.

Patients with known transudative effusions in the setting of CHF, cirrhosis, or nephrosis should not undergo pleural biopsy. Rapid separation of transudates from exudates can often be accomplished at the bedside with a refractometer of the type used to determine urine specific gravity. If malignant or tuberculous effusion is suspected, a second procedure and the attendant delay may be avoided by immediate biopsy if the fluid is shown likely to be an exudate. Balanced against this benefit, some patients will undergo biopsies when more complete analysis of pleural fluid alone would have sufficed.

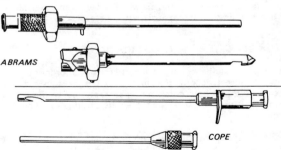

ABRAMS

COPE

Figure 10.1. Pleural biopsy needles.

After skin preparation, generous local anesthesia, and demonstrated fluid recovery at the intended site, a small skin incision is made to a depth just sufficient to penetrate the tough connective tissue plane. (A #11 blade serves nicely for this purpose.) The needle is then inserted. Considerable pressure and twisting may be required before pleural puncture is accomplished. However, insertion must be made with very firm needle control to prevent inadvertent lung puncture after sudden pleural penetration.

Two types of needle (Cope and Abrams) are in common use. Once in the pleural space, both facilitate removal of thick fluid. The Cope needle requires less force to insert but is considerably more complicated to use, provides smaller pieces, and necessitates coordinated breath-holding by the patient. The Cope biopsy hook needs frequent sharpening, and the needle is more fragile than the Abrams instrument.

Biopsies can be taken from the inferior and lateral quadrants with either instrument, but the superior quadrant is spared to avoid the neurovascular bundle.

No pleural tissue is identified in approximately 25% of samples submitted to the histology laboratory of a teaching hospital. (In experienced hands that percentage is much lower.) Yield with the Abrams needle is maximized by first inserting the instrument perpendicular to the chest wall until fluid is aspirated freely via the (side) biopsy port and then exerting gentle pressure perpendicular to the long axis of the needle in the direction of the intended biopsy. With pressure applied, the needle is carefully withdrawn until a snag is felt, and the biopsy is taken. After placement in saline or fixative, gross inspection of the pieces obtained may determine the need for another attempt. Pleural tissue appears white with an opalescent sheen, sinks in fixative, and is often attached to a shred of muscle.

SUGGESTED READINGS

1. Donohoe RF, Katz S, Matthews MJ. Pleural biopsy as an aid in the etiologic diagnosis of pleural effusion: review of the literature and report of 132 biopsies. Ann. Int. Med. 1958;48:344-62.

2. Scerbo J, Keltz H, Stone DJ. A prospective study of closed pleural biopsies. JAMA 1971;218:377-80.

3. Von Hoff DD, LiVolsi V. Diagnostic reliability of needle biopsy of the parietal pelura - a review of 272 biopsies. Am. J. Clin. Pathol. 1975;64:200-03.

Chapter 11

Chest Tubes

INDICATIONS

Chest tubes are large catheter drains placed in the pleural cavity to maintain continuous evacuation of fluid or air and to reappose the pleural surfaces. Thin fluids seldom require "tube thoracostomy," unless their rate of accumulation or potential for infection demand it. Conversely, large collections of thick fluid (blood or organizing exudates) should be drained by tube to prevent lung entrapment or loculation. Empyemas are abscesses within the pleural space that, once established, can only be eradicated by continuous drainage. Some authors advocate placement of chest tubes into large, apparently sterile parapneumonic effusions with characteristics that portend later development of empyema (low pH and glucose, and high LDH). Large effusions disadvantage the ipsilateral respiratory muscles by placing them at a high thoracic volume, mimicking hyperinflation.

A pneumothorax under tension clearly requires continuous drainage by tube thoracostomy, as does a pneumothorax caused by trauma, a pneumothorax that develops during mechanical ventilation, and a pneumothorax sufficiently large to cause dyspnea, especially in a patient with underlying cardiopulmonary disease. Most surgeons advocate chest tube placement for any large pneumothorax, even if the patient is healthy and asymptomatic. The threshold for tube placement falls progressively with increasing severity of underlying disease.

COMPLICATIONS

Pain

Many patients tolerate the severe pain of tube thoracostomy poorly and require large doses of analgesics for the first 12-48 hours following placement. Splinting related to pleurisy limits cough and deep breathing, thereby encouraging atelectasis and lung infection. Pain usually subsides to a tolerable level within 24 hours.

Subcutaneous Emphysema

Unilateral subcutaneous emphysema commonly results from tube thoracostomy, especially · when the chest tube is placed to drain air. Its mechanism of generation, however, has yet to be studied systematically. The transcutaneous incision disrupts all tissue planes. Depending on the orientation and snugness of fit between tube and skin, the potential exists for air to gain access to the subcutaneous tissue from either the pleural or skin side. It seems likely that pressure within certain subcutaneous layers is phasically subatmospheric. Air is sucked from external or undrained pleural sites during vigorous inspiration and is then trapped. Of itself, subcutaneous emphysema of this type is of no medical consequence and is usually self-limiting.

Extrapleural Placement

Lung tissue adherent to the chest wall at the site of incision may be easily ruptured and entered. Although uncommon, bronchopleural and broncho-cutaneous fistulae, as well as parenchymal damage, can ensue. Tubes are all too frequently placed into fissures, under diaphragms, and into subcutaneous tissue. These complications are more frequent when rigid trocars are employed.

Contamination of the Pleural Space

With proper sterile precautions and a well-functioning tube, this complication is surprisingly infrequent. However, if a nonfunctioning tube is left in place, contamination of reaccumulating fluid is a serious risk. Hence, a "dead tube" (not draining air or fluid in excess of 50 ml daily) should be pulled within 24-48 hours.

POINTS OF TECHNIQUE

Preparation

Inspection of a chest radiograph taken immediately prior to tube insertion is mandatory. The mobility of any fluid present should be documented by a lateral decubitus film. If the apparent fluid collection is so large as to opacify the entire hemithorax or if fluid mobility is not certain, ultrasonography or CT may confirm the presence of fluid and determine the sites of loculation.

Attempted thoracentesis should be performed at the desired site of placement to confirm the presence of fluid, especially if a question of loculation persists. Occasionally, a thickened pleural rind prevents fluid aspiration before attempted chest tube placement. In these cases, a direct operative (blunt dissection) rather than trocar approach is indicated to prevent possible lung injury.

Site of Insertion

Ideally, tubes for <u>air</u> should have the tip placed anterosuperiorly (near the apex), and tubes for fluid should be placed in the most dependent site that communicates with the fluid (posteroinferiorly). Hence, the anterior 2nd intercostal space in the mid-clavicular line is a good choice for air in a male patient with a thin chest wall. In a female patient or muscular or obese male patient, the 6th intercostal space in the mid-axillary line is suitable. (In practice, the lateral approach tends to be selected for the majority of patients, whatever their anatomy.) The 6th interspace in the mid- or posteroaxillary line is a good choice for drainage of free <u>fluid</u>, because tubes placed more posteriorly will kink and cause unnecessary discomfort.

Choice of Tube

Rubber has generally given way to nonirritating clear plastic. However, tissue irritation may be beneficial when permanent apposition of pleural surfaces is desired.

Tubes placed to drain sizable air collections should be size 20-28 French (Fr). Tubes smaller than 20 Fr tend to kink and often cannot evacuate ongoing leaks rapidly enough to ensure apposition of the pleural surfaces. Tubes placed to drain fluid should be larger: size 28-40 Fr. The largest tubes are selected for thick fluids because tubes smaller than 28 Fr occlude too easily.

Insertion

1) Two methods are commonly used to introduce the catheter into the pleural space: trocar insertion and blunt dissection.

A <u>trocar</u> is a rigid spike that bores a hole for the rigid sheath (cannula) that slides snugly over it. After the trocar is withdrawn the cannula acts as a channel into the space, through which the catheter can be inserted. In the past, the trocar and external sheath technique was used to introduce "red rubber" catheters, but in recent years internal trocars with external tubes of clear plastic have all but replaced it. (A rigid sheath is no longer used.) The modern trocar technique is quick, provides good directional guidance, and allows insertion through a small incision. However, the potential for lung puncture and intraparenchymal insertion is higher than with the blunt dissection approach.

The blunt dissection method requires a somewhat larger incision and may take a bit longer to perform. Nonetheless, because the pleural space can be directly palpated, the incidence of extrapleural placement is lower and adhesions can be detected and often lysed by finger probing.

2) An adequate number of side holes should be present in the tube to facilitate drainage of fluid and air. Too many side holes will cause the tube to kink or collapse, however. When in place, the last side hole (the "sentinal eye") should be well within the pleural space. Radiographically this sentinal eye is identified by a break in the radiopaque line that runs the length of the tube.

3) After placement, the tube can be secured with a single heavy suture that loosely approximates the upper part of the incision and anchors the tube. A second suture loosely closes the lower half. Heavy tape over dry gauze secures the tube to the chest wall to avoid painful motion.

4) Whether placed for fluid or air, the tube should be put initially to suction (15 cmH$_2$O) and the tubing connections taped carefully. At this point PA and lateral chest films must be obtained to ascertain position of the tube.

5) Generally, a tube in bad position can be pulled back but not advanced or otherwise manipulated because of the risk of pleural space contamination. If a new tube is required, it can be placed through the original incision only if the site is reprepped and no more than one hour has elapsed. If longer, a second site should be prepared.

Discontinuing the Chest Tube

Chest tubes must be removed in one quick motion, with Vaseline gauze poised to seal the wound at the instant of removal. The patient should be asked to hyperventilate immediately beforehand and to perform a Valsalva maneuver at end exhalation (FRC) as it is removed. (Slow removal will allow air to enter the thorax as the side holes are exposed to atmosphere.)

PLEURAL DRAINAGE

Tubes Placed to Drain Fluid

A chest tube placed to drain fluid must be maintained on gentle suction, or it will rapidly occlude with fibrin.

If tubing is of the opaque, flexible type, tube stripping can be done several times daily to help maintain patency. With this technique the tube is manually pinched closed near the chest and the tubing distal to the pinch point milked toward the collection bottle. Distal compression must be relieved before releasing the proximal choke point. With improper technique, very negative pressures are generated and transmitted to the pleural space during tube stripping. The significance of these very negative pressures ($\simeq$ -200 mmHg) is a bit unclear, but local trauma is one likely outcome. Sluggish tubes should never be irrigated nor any tube advanced into the chest, except during initial placement.

If the chest tube is patent and tightly applied to the chest wall, fluid in the connecting tubes should fluctuate 2.5-7.5 cmH$_2$O with each deep breath and considerably more upon coughing. This pressure swing is only a fraction of that which actually occurs during a deep breath because lung and pleural tissue plug the drainage holes as increasingly negative pressure is applied, preventing full transmission of the surface pressure fluctuation. Hence, very large pressure swings (best seen when suction is discontinued) suggest undrained air separating the tube from the lung.

As the rate of fluid accumulation slows to a minimum, gas is resorbed from the drainage tubing, which in a one-bottle system fills with liquid to levels progressively above that in the collection chamber. At the same time, the fluid level in the collection bottle fails to rise. It is then time for tube removal.

Tubes Placed to Drain Air

As a general principle, rents of the visceral pleura seal by apposition to the parietal pleura. Maintaining patency of tubes draining air without fluid is not a major problem, and smaller caliber tubes can be used. However, a single tube may not be sufficient to effect complete drainage of the pleural space, especially when the rate of air leakage is high or tube position is suboptimal.

Chest tubes that actively drain air must never be clamped longer than several minutes, or tension may develop.

After suction has been applied to juxtapose the pleural surfaces, the tube is placed to water seal after bubbling ceases. If the leak continues and the lung is not fully expanded on water seal, continuous suction is indicated. Prior to tube removal, water seal drainage should continue at least 24 hours after the lung is fully inflated and bubbling on coughing or straining has ceased.

Collection and Drainage Systems

The collection system must seal the pleural space from atmosphere yet offer minimal resistance to drainage of fluid and gas. These goals can be accomplished either with a flutter valve (which is valuable for establishing emergent decompression of a pneumothorax) or by immersing the end of the collection tube under water (water seal). Small air leaks and thin fluids drain easily with tidal fluctuations in pleural pressure and do not require the application of suction to augment the gravitational gradient. These mechanisms may not be sufficient, however, when the air leak is substantial or the fluid is proteinaceous. When a single bottle is used for both fluid collection and water seal, it becomes progressively difficult for gas and fluid to exit the chest as the fluid level builds. The effective level of suction in the one-bottle system is less than that applied by the depth of the tube tip under the fluid. Corrective adjustment can be made by raising the tube or by applying a counterbalancing suction pressure as fluid accumulates. However, a two-bottle system, where the first is used as the collection bottle and the second as the water seal, more effectively overcomes this problem.

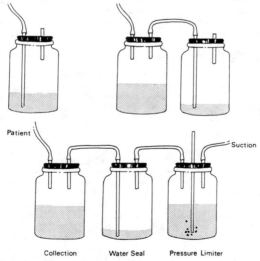

Figure 11.1. "One-, two-, and three-bottle" drainage systems.

Commonly used drainage systems provide for application of constant, controlled suction. The degree of suction can be regulated either by the vacuum pump itself (e.g., Emerson pump) or by connection of the water seal bottle to a strong vacuum source, modified to apply the desired amount of suction. This is done by leaking air into the system continuously, under a water column adjusted to the height of the desired pressure (e.g., wall suction and "3-bottle system"). The three-bottle functions can be accomplished with two bottles by adding the pressure-limiter straw to the water seal bottle. Several integrated molded plastic units are available that provide the elements of a three-bottle system in a highly portable and disposable form (e.g., Pleur-Evac). Because continuous bubbling in the suction control bottle causes evaporation, care should be taken to keep the water level carefully adjusted.

If either the one-bottle or the two-bottle system is connected to a suction source, which is then turned off, the system is closed. With a continuing air leak, pressure within the thorax may build unnoticed to produce life-threatening tension. Hence, if suction is to be discontinued, the water seal bottle must be opened to atmosphere. If suction is turned off and the pump left connected in a three-bottle system, intrathoracic pressure rises but no higher than the height of the pressure-regulating tube. Some systems recently introduced to clinical practice incorporate a "safety seal," which allows the system to decompress at a minimal positive pressure ($\simeq$ +2 cmH$_2$0).

Problems with Chest Tube Function

A chest tube can fail to effectively drain the pleural space of fluid or air for a variety of reasons. If the tube is isolated from the sites of fluid or air generation, these will not be effectively drained or decompressed. Indeed, because the flexible lung tends to "tamponade" the suction holes, such problems can develop when the tube is distant from the site of leakage, even when there are no physical seals preventing free communication in the pleural space.

Any inadvertent opening of the system proximal to the water seal can impair drainage and lead to collection of intrapleural air. When suction is applied, continuous bubbling is seen in the water seal chamber. These communications can arise at the chest tube itself if the "sentinal eye" lies outside the chest or if the skin does not seal the catheter at the site of chest entry. Connectors, bottle seals, and vents are other obvious points of concern. (Momentary clamping of the chest tube fails to stop the leak if air enters distal to the pinch point.) It should be noted that some controlled suction pumps (e.g., Emerson) continue to generate a significant vacuum at the level of pressure gauge (within the machine itself) even when widely open to atmosphere. Therefore, a substantially negative pressure reading on the pump manometer does not necessarily imply a closed system.

Two easily remediable problems commonly lead to failure of a closed system to deliver the desired level of negative pressure. Fluid evaporation from the suction control chamber of a three-bottle system lowers the vacuum level. Furthermore, with either type of controlled suction, fluid-filled dependent loops can develop in the connecting tubing. The difference in height of fluid levels between the two limbs determines the modification of applied suction.

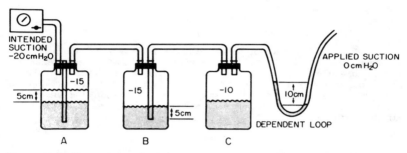

Figure 11.2. Factors contributing to failure of applied suction. A pressure of 20 cmH$_2$O applied in a three-bottle system can be attenuated by evaporation of water from the pressure-limiter bottle (A), by submersion of the water seal tube below the appropriate level of 1-2 cm (B), and by the presence of liquid in a dependent loop of connecting tubing (C).

SUGGESTED READINGS

1.   Batchelder TL, Morris KA.   Critical factors in determining adequate pleural drainage in both the operated and nonoperated chest.   Am. Surg. 1962;28:296-302.

2.   Padula RT.   Postoperative management (Chapter 8). In: Sabistan DC, and Spencer FC, eds. Surgery of the Chest. Philadelphia: Saunders, 1976:174-94.

3.   Rothberg AD, Marks KH, Maisels MJ.   Understanding the pleurevac. Pediatrics 1981;67:482-84.

Chapter 12

Pleural Sclerosis

INDICATIONS

Permanent obliteration of the space between the visceral and parietal surfaces prevents the accumulation of fluid or air. Although the most reliable methods to achieve symphysis require an operation (direct gauze abrasion, parietal pleurectomy), similar results can be achieved by tube thoracostomy and instillation of an irritating fluid that inflames the mesothelial surfaces, e.g., tetracycline. Success depends upon rigid adherence to guidelines for patient selection and technique.

Fluid

Pleural sclerosis for fluid is usually performed in symptomatic patients with rapidly recurring effusions produced by uncontrolled neoplasia. Whether repeated thoracentesis or pleural sclerosis should be done depends upon (1) the rate of fluid accumulation, (2) the severity of symptoms produced by recurring fluid, (3) the patient's tolerance for the discomfort of repeated thoracentesis, (4) the free mobility of the fluid within the chest cavity, (5) the ability of the lung to re-expand to fill the evacuated pleural space, (6) the likelihood that newly initiated therapy will control the rate of fluid accumulation without sclerosis, and (7) the projected survival of the patient.

Air

The use of pleural sclerosis by chest tube to prevent or close air leaks is somewhat controversial. There is little published evidence that it works reliably, and there has been an understandable fear that sclerosing fluid could enter the lung parenchyma via the pleural rent. However, pleural sclerosis is considered by some surgeons to offer a viable alternative to open thoracotomy, especially for patients requiring prophylactic pleural symphysis for recurrent pneumothorax and for those who are not candidates for major surgery. Indeed, a few centers have considerable experience with the use of tetracycline pleurodesis in this setting. Based on their reports, parenchymal fibrosis seems highly unlikely to present an important problem.

In the presence of an ongoing air leak, the sclerosing fluid cannot be held in contact with the pleural surfaces for the usual period. Therefore, multiple instillations may be needed to effect closure, and despite all precautions the failure rate during active air leakage is high. A prerequisite for success is that the inflamed pleural surfaces can be held in contact to allow tissue bridges to form. Patients with large air leaks are poor candidates. An unsuccessful attempt may produce patchy adhesions that make later surgery difficult. Nevertheless, occasional patients who continue to leak air despite weeks of suction either refuse surgery or cannot withstand thoracotomy. In these instances, placement of a new tube and attempted pleural sclerosis seems reasonable if the patient is watched closely during the initial period of tube clamping.

COMPLICATIONS

Bringing inflamed pleural surfaces into direct contact can cause extreme pain, especially with a large thoracostomy tube in place. Pain is most intense during the initial period following tetracycline instillation. Adding 200 mg of lidocaine to the sclerosing solution may help temporarily. Pleurodesis is performed under general anesthesia in some centers. "Vasovagal" reactions are not uncommon. Prophylactic atropine may be helpful.

Low-grade fever develops frequently and persists for 24-48 hours. Some agents, such as quinacrine, cause particularly intense inflammation and pyrexia.

Antineoplastic agents, such as nitrogen mustard, were among the earliest agents used for treatment of pleural malignancy. Occasionally, neutropenia related to systemic absorption occurred. Since these chemotherapeutic drugs are no more effective than less toxic agents, they are seldom used currently.

POINTS OF TECHNIQUE

Because success depends upon the ability to reappose diffusely inflamed pleural surfaces, the lung must be mobile (neither encased by a visceral pleural rind nor kept from inflating by blockage of a central bronchus). Furthermore, an effective concentration of sclerosing liquid must reach all pleural surfaces. Loculations and undrained fluid pockets impede dispersion and dilute the solution, respectively.

A functioning tube thoracostomy must effectively drain the pleural space. Injection into a preexisting chest tube may cause infection and is not recommended. Instillation of sclerosing solution after thoracentesis (without thoracostomy) seldom works because the exudate caused by the reaction itself pushes the pleural surfaces apart. Attempting sclerosis with undrained fluid present is futile.

Quinacrine (600-800 mg) in 30 ml 0.9 N saline, talc (10 gm of sterile, aerated powder suspended in 250 ml of 0.9 N saline), and tetracycline (25 mg/kg in a 50 ml volume) are probably equally effective if instilled properly. Tetracycline is perhaps the best choice, due to its availability and patient tolerance.   Animal experiments indicate that high concentrations of tetracycline are required for the best results. Hence, 25 mg/kg tetracycline in 40 ml 0.9 N saline and 10 ml of 2% lidocaine is a rational choice.

Sequence

Fluid

1. Determine radiographically whether the lung can move away from the chest wall with upright and bilateral decubitus films. A small diagnostic pneumothorax may be helpful if doubt exists.

2. Insert a large (e.g., 36 Fr) chest tube with multiple side holes by the blunt dissection technique. Using the finger, probe the pleural space for adhesions before insertion. Connect the tube to suction.

3. Drain the pleural space of all fluid by rolling the recumbent patient into all four quadrants, changing every 2-3 minutes. Confirm dryness by repeat chest film.

4. Discontinue suction and inject tetracycline solution together with 100-200 ml of air, creating a small pneumothorax to facilitate distribution of sclerosing liquid.

5. To coat all pleural surfaces, turn the recumbent patient into supine, prone, lateral, and Trendelenburg positions, changing every 2-3 minutes.

6. Return the patient to the supine, prone, and both lateral positions for 30 minutes each, with the tube clamped. Then resume suction (-15 cmH$_2$0).

7. Pull the tube when drainage has stopped for 24 hours.

Air

The procedure for pleurodesis of an air leak is similar. However, if the air leak is sizable, tube clamping must be brief, if attempted at all. Multiple (2-3) instillations of sclerosing fluid over a several day period may help to improve the generally lower success rate with this procedure.

SUGGESTED READINGS

1. Austin EH, Flye MW. The treatment of recurrent malignant pleural effusion. Ann. Thorac. Surg. 1979;28:190-203.

2. Good JT, Sahn SA. Intrapleural therapy with tetracycline in malignant pleural effusions. Chest 1978;74:602.

3. Larrieu AJ, et al. Intrapleural instillation of quinacrine for treatment of recurrent spontaneous pneumothorax. Ann. Thorac. Surg. 1979;28:146-50.

4. Light RW. Pleural Diseases. Philadelphia: Lea and Febiger, 1983.

5. Wallach HW. Intrapleural tetracycline for malignant pleural effusions. Chest 1975;68:510-12.

Chapter 13

Collection and Interpretation of Sputum Specimens

COLLECTION METHODS

Obtaining the Specimen

Sputum may provide clues to infection, neoplasia, or allergy. The deepest specimens are most often recovered in the early morning and after bronchoscopy. Since the specimen must pass the oropharynx, dentures should be removed and the mouth rinsed several times with tap water beforehand to reduce contamination. Patients with loose secretions but who will not spontaneously raise sputum can often be induced to expectorate by an irritating aerosol of distilled water or hypertonic saline. A heated ultrasonic nebulizer is a particularly effective means of delivery. Chest percussion and postural drainage are also useful measures. If these methods fail, nasotracheal suctioning may be effective. None of these techniques will recover secretions if the cough is dry.

In patients with suspected active tuberculosis but no sputum, early-morning gastric aspirates for culture may be helpful because sputum swallowed overnight remains in the stomach for a short time after waking. (Acid-fast stains are not done because nonpathogenic acid-fast bacteria are often resident there and confound interpretation.) However, the ease and precision of fiberoptic biopsy and lavage, together with its potential for enabling rapid histologic diagnosis, have all but rendered gastric aspirates obsolescent.

Acceptable specimens for anaerobic culture are obtained by transtracheal aspiration, thoracentesis, or direct lung puncture. Specimens for viral culture are best collected by having the patient gargle and expectorate nutrient broth or by wiping the nasal or oral pharynx and transporting the swab in viral culture medium, as directed by the microbiology laboratory. If unusual pathogens are suspected, contact the laboratory before collection to comply with special requirements.

A tumor in a central bronchus sheds cells sporadically into coughed sputum. In such cases, approximately 40% of deep cough specimens for sputum cytology show evidence of the underlying neoplasm and the percentage of positive diagnoses improves noticeably when at least four specimens are taken at separate times. Specimens obtained after bronchoscopy have higher yield. Peripheral lung tumors and tumors metastatic to the lung have a smaller chance of being detected by cytology of expectorated sputum, in part because many such neoplasms grow or seed in extrabronchial sites. Successful identification of the cell of origin depends heavily on tumor type and degree of differentiation, as well as on the skill of the cytologist. Sputum recovered from patients with active inflammation is suboptimal for cytological examination because inflammation may cause bizarre cellular changes resembling malignancy.

Fixation of sputum for cytological purposes should be done immediately (without air drying) by having the patient expectorate directly into a wide-mouthed jar containing 70% ethanol. (Spreading the fresh specimen thinly onto a glass slide with rapid immersion in Pap fixative is an alternate technique.)

TRANSPORT

If the specimen is to be cultured for aerobic bacteria, it must be brought quickly to the laboratory before overgrowth of mouth organisms has occurred or fastidious pathogens die. Anaerobic cultures must be transported in an airtight container (such as a capped syringe) and plated immediately. Tuberculosis bacilli are robust and can withstand 24-48 hours of storage at room temperature without notable consequence.

If transport must be delayed, refrigeration will forestall significant overgrowth for several hours. In the laboratory, washing the specimen several times with saline and then discarding the supernatant will reduce contamination with oral flora. (Nonviscid saliva and its organisms are discarded with the saline.)

EXAMINATION

Site of Origin

Expectorated material can originate from nasal passages, the oropharynx, or the lower airway. (Occasionally gastric contents are admixed.)

Watching the patient produce the sample often indicates its origin. Examination of the gross specimen may reveal other clues. Foamy, clear material usually represents salivary or nasal secretions. Ordinarily, sputum from patients with chronic bronchitis is mucoid and cloudy. Change in color indicates acute infection or allergic inflammation. Purulent material is usually produced in the sinuses or lung but may result from allergy or infection in either area. Very adhesive sputum is likely to be allergic in origin.

Feculent odors suggest anaerobic infection, but many anaerobic infections do not produce an offensive odor. Fresh blood from the lung is always bright red. Brown pigment indicates altered hemoglobin and characterizes a nonacute pulmonary hemorrhage or blood altered by gastric acid. Sputum with a three-layered appearance suggests stagnation of purulent secretions within the lung and is recovered most often with lung abscess or bronchiectasis.

Microscopy of the Unstained Specimen

An unrefrigerated sputum specimen begins to autodigest within minutes. A cooled specimen will retain cellular integrity for 24 hours or longer. Examination of unstained sputum allows separation of allergic and infectious causes for respiratory distress, especially among patients with exacerbations of chronic airflow obstruction. Furthermore, the "quality" of a specimen and its suitability for culture may be judged within minutes.

To perform microscopy, a strand or plug is teased from the specimen and placed on a slide. (An equal amount of buffered crystal violet may be added to enhance contrast and aid cell identification, if desired.) A cover slip is added and the specimen is examined under oil. The structures observed are contaminating oropharyngeal cells, cells originating from lung tissue, inflammatory cells, and noncellular elements. The presence of bronchial epithelial cells, alveolar macrophages, or polymorphonuclear leukocytes, together with a paucity of squamous cells, indicates that the specimen originated within the lung and suggests suitability for culture. The cellular content of normal secretions is mainly bronchial epithelium (basal, ciliated, and goblet cells). Unusual forms of shed bronchial epithelium (creola bodies) are seen in profusion in viral illnesses. Alveolar macrophages tend to appear only after infection is well established or resolving.

A concentration of eosinophils in the sputum exceeding 5% suggests the existence of an active allergic component. Eosinophils can be distinguished readily from polymorphonuclear leukocytes by the presence of large granules. Eosinophils constitute 5-90% of all cells in sputum from asthmatics, the concentration varying with acuteness and steroid treatment. Wright's stain enhances their recognition. Purulence caused by eosinophilia suggests that corticosteroids, not antibiotics, are indicated. Sputum eosinophilia may be the only indication that the inflammation is allergic in origin. Superimposed infection and corticosteroid therapy can cause eosinophils to disappear from the sputum. Other findings that indicate ongoing allergic bronchitis are Charcot-Leyden crystals and Curschmann spirals.

Examination for Microbes

Gram Stain

The Gram stain is an essential complement to culture. This test not only allows sound judgment to be made as to the presence of infection and adequacy of the specimen for culture but also provides a method for choosing antibiotics appropriately before culture results are known. If several organisms grow up in culture, the initial Gram stain may provide the best indication of the pathogen responsible for illness. The Gram stain may be the only way to diagnose disease due to fastidious organisms, such as pneumococci and anaerobes. The absence of Gram-stainable bacteria in purulent sputum suggests viral, mycoplasmal, mycobacterial, and certain fungal pathogens. Legionella species tend to be Gram negative but can be missed entirely on a standard smear. Tuberculosis bacilli and Nocardia stain weakly Gram positive, and Candida stains strongly positive.

Many microbiology laboratories grade the quality of sputum specimens on a simple scale to express the degree of confidence placed in its interpretation and culture. Squamous epithelial cells in numbers greater than 10 per low power (10x) field suggest an upper airway origin and should be discarded in favor of a deeper specimen. During active inflammation, leukocytes in a "good" specimen should be at least 7-10 times as plentiful as squamous cells. Mucous threads may be evident. If there are fewer than 3-5 polys per high power field (oil), the area surveyed for organisms probably did not originate in an area of intense inflammation. Stain of another likely looking droplet should be prepared if no suitable areas are found. Most polymorphonuclear leukocytes should appear intact in fresh sputum specimens. If not, the specimen may be old and overgrown.

If a bacterial organism is responsible for inflammation, it should predominate. (Cultures with significant growth of more than four organisms suggest oropharyngeal contamination.) Bacteria should be present in approximately the same numbers as polys. They are described as rare to 4+, depending on whether fewer than 1 per 5 oil immersion fields to greater than 50 per oil immersion field are seen. Intracellular organisms indicate ingestion by polys of opsonized bacteria, suggesting both that the organism is important and that the inflammation is several days old. Wright and Giemsa stains may highlight intracellular organisms to advantage.

Although nondescript by Gram stain, Legionella deserves special mention, in that direct fluorescent antibody staining techniques may hold the best chance of early detection.

Stains for Mycobacteria

Acid-fast mycobacteria take up the Ziehl-Neelsen stain, tinting red against a blue background. Typical m. TB stains unevenly, with a tendency toward accumulation of stain at the poles and a beaded appearance. The Kenyoun stain is quicker but somewhat less reliable. Since relatively few mycobacteria are usually present, a slide must be examined for longer than 15 minutes before calling it negative. False positives commonly result from atypical mycobacteria originating in chronically diseased lungs (or even in the laboratory reagents).

Fluorochrome dyes (auramine, rhodamine) require a special microscope for interpretation but cause organisms to stand out strikingly to aid rapid identification. Unfortunately, false positives occur more often than with the Ziehl-Neelsen stain.

Fungal Organisms

As a rule, most fungal pathogens are difficult to identify in expectorated sputum. When present, different fungi are best identified by a variety of staining techniques. Candida species are highlighted well by Gram stain, taking on a strongly Gram-positive character. Blastomycosis (and crypto-coccosis) is often best identified by sputum cytology, not by standard microbiologic methods. Histoplasmosis, coccidioidomycosis, aspergillus, and mucor show up best with PAS or methenamine silver staining. A simple KOH prep, in which heated 10% KOH is used to digest cellular material, may allow for visual isolation of yeast or branching filaments.

SUGGESTED READINGS

1. Chodosh S. Examination of sputum cells. N. Engl. J. Med. 1970;282:854-57.

2. Epstein RL. Constituents of sputum: a simple method. Ann. Intern. Med. 1972;77:259-65.

3. Epstein RL, Jain BP. Sputum examination (Chapter 6). In: Fishman AP, ed. Pulmonary Diseases and Disorders. New York: McGraw Hill, 1980:103-10.

4. Johnston WW, Frable WJ. The cytopathology of the respiratory tract: a review. Am. J. Pathol. 1976;84:372-414.

5. Scharf SM, Heimer D. Laboratory evaluation of patients with respiratory disease (Chapter 11). In: Baum GL, Wolinsky E, eds. Textbook of Pulmonary Diseases (3rd Edition). Boston: Little Brown, 1983:235-48.

Chapter 14

Transtracheal Aspiration

INDICATIONS

Expectorated samples are frequently suboptimal for identification of pneumonic pathogens. The respiratory tract is usually sterile below the larynx, except in patients with chronic bronchopulmonary infections. Mouth flora contaminate expectorated sputum so that the recovery of pathogenic organisms does not necessarily indicate lower tract involvement. The rich oropharyngeal growth of anaerobes renders expectorated sputum worthless for culture of these organisms. All too frequently, cooperative patients provide only saliva for examination or cannot raise pulmonary secretions. Obtunded and uncooperative patients do not expectorate at all.

Transtracheal aspiration (TA) via needle puncture of the cricothyroid membrane provides a highly satisfactory specimen of pulmonary secretions. Samples are quite sensitive and specific in detecting the responsible bacterial pathogens. Even a negative TA has differential diagnostic value; if organisms are neither stained nor cultured, the possibility of virus, legionella, mycoplasma, or mycobacteria is strengthened.

Unfortunately, in unpracticed hands TA often causes significant morbidity and therefore should not be performed indiscriminately. Perhaps the majority of patients can produce satisfactory deep cough specimens. Furthermore, community-acquired pneumonia in otherwise healthy adults responds rather predictably to penicillin, cephalosporin, or erythromycin, obviating the necessity of a precise bacteriologic diagnosis. However, TA should be considered if a seriously ill patient expectorates material laden with Gram-negative organisms, yeast, or clumps of apparent staphylococci. These findings suggest that routine antibiotics, doses, and durations of treatment are inappropriate.

The pharynx of many hospitalized patients, especially those requiring intensive care, colonizes with unusual organisms, which later may be aspirated to cause pneumonia. Unless the expectorated sample is satisfactory, as judged by gross and microscopic characteristics (see p. 77), TA is appropriate. The more seriously ill the patient, the more important precise bacteriologic diagnosis becomes. Apparent bacterial pneumonia in a patient with compromised host defenses should prompt consideration of TA, because such infections are often caused by Gram-negative organisms with unusual antibiotic susceptibility patterns and particular virulence for this population. Fungi may also be recovered. Suspected anaerobic pneumonia should be confirmed. Transthoracic needle aspiration and sampling of the parenchyma with a sheathed catheter at bronchoscopy are viable alternative procedures to TA for physicians experienced in their use.

Contraindications: This procedure cannot be performed safely in patients with agitation, severe coughing, significant clotting deficiencies, recent myocardial infarction, hemodynamic instability, uncorrected hypoxemia, or ongoing asthma. If nasotracheal suctioning has previously been performed within 6 hours, the lower airway must be considered contaminated and the results of TA suspect.

COMPLICATIONS

TA-induced intratracheal or peritracheal hemorrhage, hypoxemia, arrhythmias, vasovagal reactions, subcutaneous emphysema, bronchospasm, and angina pectoris are not rare. Although reported, gastric aspiration, upper airway obstruction (due to submucosal hematoma or laryngospasm), pneumothorax, myocardial infarction, and sudden death are highly unusual.

POINTS OF TECHNIQUE

Assess platelets, protime, PTT, PaO_2, and cardiopulmonary status beforehand. Administer 0.8-1.2 mg atropine IM prior to procedure. Monitor cardiac rhythm by electrocardiogram. Administer sufficient supplemental oxygen to raise arterial saturation to at least 95%. Have intubation tray, endotracheal suction equipment, and emergency drug box at bedside for use as needed.

After local anesthesia and sedation are achieved, puncture the cricothyroid membrane just above the cricoid cartilage, twist the needle to direct the bevel caudally, and insert the intraluminal catheter with the needle slightly inclined inferiorly. Withdraw the needle completely from the trachea as the catheter is advanced. (To avoid shearing, never withdraw the catheter through the needle.) When coughing begins, attempt to aspirate. If no material enters the syringe, aspirate again after injecting 5-10 ml of non-bacteriostatic saline.

Withdraw the catheter and apply firm pressure for 5-10 minutes to minimize bleeding and subcutaneous emphysema. Reexamine and observe the patient closely for several hours afterward. Vigorous coughing should be discouraged for 12-24 hours postprocedure.

SUGGESTED READINGS

1. Bartlett JG. Diagnostic accuracy of transtracheal aspiration bacteriologic studies. Am. Rev. Respir. Dis. 1977;115:777-82.

2. Hahn HH, Beaty HN. Transtracheal aspiration in the evaluation of patients with pneumonia. Ann. Intern. Med. 1970;72:183-87.

3. Irwin RS, Pratter MR. Transtracheal aspiration procedure: a protocol. Chest 1981;79:245-47.

4. Pratter MR, Irwin RS. Transtracheal aspiration: guidelines for safety. Chest 1979;76:518-20.

5. Spencer CD, Beaty HN. Complications of transtracheal aspiration. N. Engl. J. Med. 1972;286:304-06.

Chapter 15

Endotracheal Intubation

INDICATIONS

Indications for endotracheal intubation include:

(1) need for assisted ventilation or high levels of inspired oxygen
(2) airway protection against aspiration
(3) clearance of secretions retained in central airways
(4) upper airway obstruction

Endotracheal tubes should be removed as soon as the indication for their continued presence abates. All such tubes bypass the mechanical defenses of the upper airway against infection, grossly contaminate the lower airways, and severely hamper effective coughing. Despite advances in cuff design and construction materials, all tubes have the potential of causing permanent laryngeal and tracheal injury, and none completely protect the lungs against aspiration of fluids and oropharyngeal secretions.

Tracheal intubation can be achieved via nasal, oral, and cervical routes. Orotracheal tubes are generally easier to insert and larger than nasotracheal tubes. Ease of insertion makes them the airway of choice in an emergency. Larger size improves airway resistance and secretion management and allows passage of a fiberoptic bronchoscope, if the need arises. However, they are less stable, less comfortable, and impair swallowing to a greater extent than nasotracheal tubes. In addition, maintenance of orpharyngeal hygiene is difficult. Conventional orotracheal intubation often cannot or should not be performed in patients with limited neck mobility. The recent introduction of the illuminated stylet makes feasible orotracheal intubations in patients for whom the larynx cannot be directly visualized and for those in whom the neck must be maintained in a neutral position (cervical trauma, severe rheumatoid arthritis, etc.).

Nasotracheal tubes have relatively high resistance compared with other tubes of similar diameter because they are long, kink easily, and frequently encrust with secretions. Furthermore, the nares do not admit tubes as large as those that the larynx will accept comfortably. Nasotracheal tubes are more difficult to insert and after several days may cause purulent nasal discharge or sinusitis.

Tracheostomy provides maximal comfort (potentially allowing the patient to eat and talk), allows excellent secretion management, minimizes airway resistance and anatomic dead space, and eliminates the risk of laryngeal injury. Tracheostomy also allows effective spontaneous cough if PEEP is not required. However, tracheostomies have the highest associated risk of serious complications (bleeding, stenosis), and the incidence of post-extubation swallowing difficulty and aspiration is also highest with this route. Unless carried out emergently for acute upper airway obstruction, tracheostomy should always be performed over an oral or nasal tube in an operating suite.

COMPLICATIONS

Insertion Trauma

Inexpert placement of an endotracheal tube may injure laryngeal, nasal, and pharyngeal tissues or cause dental trauma.

Hypoxemia / Ischemia

Patients who require supplemental oxygen for adequate gas exchange often undergo prolonged exposure to room air during intubation, with consequent desaturation of arterial blood. Although this risk is minimized to some extent by "preoxygenation" with several deep breaths of oxygen, the quantity of oxygen stored in this way is quickly depleted if the patient washes it from the lungs by breathing deeply (see p. 24). If difficulty is encountered, the attempt should not be prolonged beyond 30 seconds before "re-oxygenating." This guideline can be relaxed somewhat if paralytic drugs are used to establish apnea. Nasal prongs set to deliver 6 liters of oxygen can provide some oxygen supplementation during insertion.

Depletion of the oxygen reservoir can be prevented by administration of a rapid-acting hypnotic (e.g., thiopental 25-100 mg IV) followed by succinyl-choline (1 mg/kg) to induce temporary paralysis. (If the patient is at risk for cardiac instability, vecuronium, although somewhat longer acting, is perhaps a safer choice.) This apneic intubation technique also facilitates cannulation of the larynx, shortens the time without ventilation, and lessens the hazards of laryngospasm and insertion trauma. Although apneic intubation is the preferred technique in difficult cases, the administration of sedatives and muscle relaxants is not without risk in this setting. Relaxation of the musculature of the upper airway may cause partial or complete upper airway obstruction if measures are not taken to keep the passage open. Rarely, succinylcholine can induce the syndrome of "malignant hyperpyrexia" - a life-threatening problem, treatable with dantrolene.

Cessation of cardiopulmonary resuscitation efforts while a desperate attempt is made to "secure the airway" poses an even greater risk than apnea. Ischemia is less well tolerated than hypoxia alone. Cardiac compression should not be interrupted for longer than 10-15 seconds, especially if the lungs can be effectively ventilated by mask without intubation.

In general, the blind nasotracheal approach should not be attempted during emergent intubation of a deteriorating patient because of the uncertain length of time required to secure the airway. When semiemergent placement of a nasal tube is required, fiberoptic bronchoscopy often facilitates intubation.

Gastric Aspiration

Stimulation of the oropharynx frequently causes reflex vomiting of gastric contents, especially when the stomach has been distended by prolonged mask insufflation. Gentle cricothyroid pressure from the start of mask ventilation until the tube is placed will help seal the esophagus against air entry. If feasible, evacuation of the stomach contents before the intubation attempt will limit this risk.

Esophageal Intubation

Although usually of little consequence, esophageal intubation is potentially disastrous if unrecognized. Look for expansion of the upper chest to indicate that air enters the lungs and listen for rapid exhalation of air through the tube. Quickly auscultate the lung fields and abdomen during insufflation. If uncertainty continues, extubate, reoxygenate, and try again. Theoretically, esophageal intubation should not happen if the intubator visualizes the cords as the tube passes through them. Again, use of a lighted stylet permits transcutaneous visualization of the tube tip as it passes the larynx and minimizes the risk of this complication.

Laryngospasm

Reflex laryngospasm can prevent passage of the endotracheal tube and severely limit ventilation. Rather than attempt forceful intubation, losing valuable time and producing laryngeal trauma, ventilate with oxygen by mask.

Spasm usually subsides spontaneously within seconds. However, if adequate ventilation cannot be achieved and the situation becomes urgent, succinylcholine (1 mg/kg, IV) will release the spasm. Prior use of a topical anesthetic (lidocaine, 4%) will minimize the risk.

Bronchospasm

Tube placement often triggers the irritant receptors that line the upper airway, producing cough and bronchospasm. In susceptible patients, an asthmatic attack may result. Irritant receptors stop firing shortly after tube placement in most cases, unless the tip of the tube rests low enough to touch the carina. Coughing is difficult to arrest, but an endotracheal lidocaine bolus (5 ml of 2%) may help. In addition to an aminophylline infusion, nebulized atropine (2 mg) is a good choice for bronchospasm but will not alleviate coughing.

Right Main Bronchus Intubation

There is a natural tendency to place endotracheal tubes too low, especially in emergent situations. The right main bronchus is less sharply angulated from the trachea than is the left and will be entered in 90% of such placements. As a consequence, the underventilated left lung may collapse rapidly, especially if previously ventilated with oxygen. The right upper lobe orifice may also be occluded, causing an additional problem. Although comparative auscultation is helpful, breath sounds are often surprisingly well transmitted to an underventilated lung, giving misleading information.

Endotracheal tubes should be advanced a maximum of 2.5-5.0 cm beyond the point at which the tube cuff is seen to pass the cords. Use of a lighted stylet facilitates tip localization to the appropriate level. As a general rule, 22 cm at the 2nd molar will approximate the proper position in an average-size adult. A postprocedure chest film is necessary to check position. A generous distance between tube tip and main carina must be allowed, since the tube tip can move 2 cm toward the carina with neck flexion, 2 cm away from the carina with neck extension, and 1 cm away with lateral rotation of the head.

POINTS OF TECHNIQUE

Oral Intubation

Apart from being well prepared for emergent developments, perhaps the most important thing for the physician to do is to relax. After clearing the airway of debris, dislodge the base of the tongue from the retropharynx by lifting at the angles of the jaw and place an oropharyngeal airway to maintain the channel. Position the patient with the head (not shoulders) resting on a thin pillow or a doubly folded towel. The optimal position is with the neck flexed and the head strongly extended. Once this is done, the patient can generally be ventilated by mask without difficulty until the tube is inserted. Bag insufflations should be gentle and frequent rather than forceful and slow.

If tube placement is not emergent, premedicate an alert patient with atropine (0.8 mg IM) and atomize lidocaine (4%) as the patient pants to deposit most of the drug on the larynx and upper airway.

Agitated or seriously hypoxic patients should be sedated quickly and paralyzed (apneic intubation technique, p. 84).

For an average-size male, a 9.0-mm (internal diameter) tube and, for a female, an 8.0-mm tube are good sizes to try first. Choose the largest tube that will easily pass the cords.

A curved laryngoscope blade is directed anterior to the epiglottis. Straight blade instruments are inserted immediately posterior to the epiglottis and allow a better view of the cords. Both instruments should be applied to lift the entire jaw upward to expose the larynx. Neither instrument should use the teeth as a fulcrum for leverage to expose the glottis.

During intubation, firm cricothryoid pressure helps to bring the cords into view and to seal the esophagus.

A flexible stylet can be used to direct the tip of the tube ventrally, into a glottic opening that cannot be completely visualized. Illuminated stylets are particularly helpful for this purpose. When directed properly, the point of light is easily viewed through the thin tissue of the anterior trachea and skin. To avoid laryngeal trauma, care must be taken to ensure that the stylet does not project beyond the tip of the tube.

After placement, inflate the cuff with the minimum volume that seals without leakage under positive pressure. A standard orotracheal tube is best anchored by a continuous single band of tape wrapped circumferentially around the neck and secured to the tube and bite block at both ends.

Flexible fiberoptic instruments (bronchoscope, laryngoscope) can be used to excellent advantage when intubating a difficult patient or one with limited neck mobility. This is of particular importance in patients with ankylosing spondylitis or rheumatoid arthritis who have an increased risk of C_1 - C_2

subluxation with neck extension. Supplemental oxygen need not be interrupted if the fiberscope is inserted through a perforated T-piece adapter attached to the endotracheal tube.

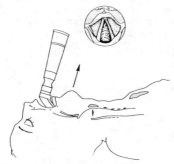

Figure 15.1. Orotracheal intubation. To align glottis, pharynx, and oral cavity, the neck is flexed and the head extended. The laryngoscope lifts the tongue and lower jaw away from the posterior pharynx by a motion directed perpendicular to the oroglottic axis.

Extubation

Administer oxygen by nasal prongs and clear both the trachea and the oropharynx of secretions by suction before deflating the cuff. After a deep inspiration the tube should be pulled quickly as the patient rapidly exhales from total lung capacity (usually producing sputum by the effort). Post-extubation stridor may occur due to laryngospasm or supraglottic or subglottic edema. This usually abates within the first 6-24 hours, but such patients must be observed especially carefully to assess the need for urgent reintubation.

SUGGESTED READINGS

1. Salem MR, Mathrabhutham M, Bennett EJ. Difficult intubation. N. Engl. J. Med. 1976;295:879-81.

2. Selwyn AS. Endotracheal Intubation (Chapter 17). In: Vander Salm TJ, ed. Atlas of Bedside Procedures. Boston: Little Brown, 1979:159-68.

3. Stauffer JL, Silvestri RC. Complications of endotracheal intubation in tracheostomy and artificial airways. Respiratory Care 1982;27:417-34.

Chapter 16

Prescribing Respiratory Therapy

Few hospital services are as valuable to patient care or as subject to overutilization as respiratory therapy (RT). In the desire to do the maximum possible for the patient, RT has often been applied indiscriminately, at substantial discomfort, morbidity, and financial cost for the patient. Unlike the past, respiratory care services are now under extraordinary pressure to become optimally cost-effective, as hospitals immerse in the environment of prospective payment. It is the physician who determines the treatment type and intensity. Understanding the indications and contraindications for RT procedures is vital to appropriate patient management.

PROCEDURES: ASSISTED COUGHING

Because spontaneous forceful coughing is by far the most effective method of clearing the airway, encouraging the reluctant patient to cough is among the most valuable services a therapist provides. Gentle external vibration of the cricoid cartilage may stimulate cough, as may deep breathing alone in patients with airways irritated by edema or inflammation. An ultrasonic aerosol of distilled water or saline is often effective when other methods fail, but must be administered cautiously (see p. 100).

Nasotracheal suctioning serves two purposes: to stimulate the coughing efforts that bring distal secretions to central airways and to aspirate secretions retained in the central bronchi. Traumatic and uncomfortable, its use should be minimized, especially in patients with heart disease. Associated vagal stimulation and hypoxemia can be arrhythmogenic. Cooperative patients with cuffless or fenestrated tracheostomies can be taught to cough effectively by momentarily occluding the tube orifice as a forceful effort is made against a closed glottis. Pressure can then build to a level sufficient to expel secretions through the pharynx. Many patients can be assisted by applying a pillow to splint painful areas of the abdomen or chest. Exhalation pressure can be increased in patients with quadriplegia by abdominal compression coordinated with the patient's spontaneous efforts.

DEEP BREATHING

Healthy individuals spontaneously take breaths 2-3 times greater than the normal tidal depth 8-10 times per hour. Many influences, including sedatives, coma, and thoracoabdominal surgery, abolish this pattern, encouraging atelectasis and secretion retention. Although the main purpose of deep breathing ("hyperinflation") is to restore prophylactic lung stretching, stimulation of a productive cough is a side benefit for some patients.

Useful deep breathing starts from FRC, ends at TLC, and sustains inflation at a high lung volume for several seconds. Maneuvers that encourage exhalation rather than inhalation actually may be counterproductive. Thus, "blow-bottles," which ask the patient to transfer fluid from one bottle to another by positive pressure, are only helpful if the lung is stretched to a high volume and the exhalation effort ceases at FRC. Few patients follow these guidelines but instead operate at lower, less painful lung volumes.

Proper positioning of the patient is perhaps the most effective means of maintaining lung volume. In moving from the supine to the upright posture, lung volume may increase 500-1000 ml, a volume increase equivalent to 5-10 cmH_2O PEEP! Turning the bedridden patient side-to-side at frequent intervals achieves involuntary distension and encourages gravitational drainage of the uppermost lung, while improving perfusion and ventilation of the lower lung. Changing position in patients with unilateral disease may have notable effects on both gas exchange and secretion clearance. Turning is especially important for patients immobilized by trauma, sedation, or paralysis.

INCENTIVE SPIROMETRY, IPPB, and CPAP

These methods are used to encourage deep breathing and to maintain a higher lung volume. An incentive spirometer is a device that gives a visual indication of whether the inhalation effort is satisfactory. The frequency of deep breathing may also be tabulated. Unlike IPPB, an incentive spirometer can be used by the cooperative, unattended patient. Furthermore, the distribution of ventilation tends to be more uniform than with IPPB. Although some devices measure inspiratory flow rate, it is better to measure inhaled volume. Units that reward flow are prone to misuse, since a high inspiratory flow rate can be achieved by a low-amplitude, unsustained effort begun at a low lung volume.

IPPB is generally overprescribed. However, a valid use is to provide deep breaths to a cooperative patient otherwise too weak to inhale a similar volume. (Effective IPPB is difficult to deliver to an uncooperative patient.) Unaccompanied by an increase in lung volume, positive pressure alone does little to forestall or reverse atelectasis. Volume-cycled ventilators deliver the set volume unless leakage occurs but, due to their lack of portability and cost, are not often used for this purpose. Instead, pressure-limited machines are generally used. Although convenient, their purpose can be easily circumvented by expiratory muscle contraction or high impedance to chest inflation. Therefore, the volume administered should be measured and compared against the spontaneous inspiratory capacity. Treatments should be terminated if the IPPB-delivered breath does not exceed the spontaneous inspiratory capacity at a safe level of pressure (20-30 cmH$_2$O). IPPB may force air into the esophagus, resulting in gastric distension and discomfort. Contraindications to IPPB include pneumothorax, mediastinal or subcutaneous emphysema, cardiovascular insufficiency, tracheoesophageal fistula, and recent gastrectomy.

Intermittent use of CPAP applied by a tight-fitting mask has been reported to be as successful as these other methods in improving gas exchange. Its primary advantages are that little patient cooperation or personnel time are required and that the increment in lung volume is sustained, improving efficacy. The value of CPAP in therapy has yet to be settled, however.

BRONCHODILATOR ADMINISTRATION

Another reasonable use of IPPB is to administer an aerosolized bronchodilator to a nonintubated patient who cannot breathe deeply. In stronger, cooperative patients, a compressor-driven nebulizer provides a more effective method. Although suboptimal, a nebulizer used with a mouthpiece or simple face mask can be used to deposit a small amount of drug on the airways if no other method is feasible. In general, metered-dose cannisters do not deliver the intended dosage unless the patient is capable of coordinating the puff with the breathing cycle or a spacing chamber attachment is used. The latter is a very promising technique for marginally cooperative or maladroit hospitalized patients and may be comparable in efficacy to the compressor-driven method. If the patient is mechanically ventilated, medication delivery is accomplished by nebulization into the circuit. By any of these methods, the dose should be given by multiple inhalations over a 5-15 minute period to maximize its effect.

CHEST PERCUSSION AND POSTURAL DRAINAGE (PHYSIOTHERAPY, CPT)

The objectives of chest percussion and postural drainage are to dislodge retained secretions from peripheral airways and to aid clearance of sputum retained in the central airways. Vibration or hand percussion is done for 5-15 minutes with the involved segment(s) in the position of best gravitational drainage, and the postural drainage position is maintained for an additional 5-15 minutes afterward. For the optimal result, bronchodilator administration should precede CPT and deep breathing, and coughing should be encouraged before, during, and after the 10-15 minutes of posturing. Patients likely to benefit from this treatment are those who retain secretions because of impaired clearance mechanics (e.g., airflow obstruction, neuromuscular weakness, or postoperative pain). CPT is of demonstrated benefit in patients with acute lobar atelectasis. It is not surprising that studies of CPT's efficacy in patients who retain a vigorous cough have shown little benefit. It may well be helpful for patients with pneumonia who are unable to clear secretions pooled in the central airways. Chest physiotherapy is appropriate in the intensive care setting, provided that thoracic incisions, tubes, position limitation, rib fractures, hypotension, or other mechanical impediments do not contraindicate its use.

Occasional patients experience dyspnea during chest physiotherapy, presumably due to increased venous return, positional hypoxemia, or increased work of breathing or decreased muscular efficiency in head-dependent positions. Available data warrant prophylactic oxygen supplementation during and shortly following treatment.

ENDOTRACHEAL SUCTIONING

The trachea may be suctioned to provide a sputum specimen in an uncooperative or debilitated patient or to clear the central airway of secretions. Inherently traumatic, hazardous, and less effective than a productive cough, tracheal suctioning should only be done when a sputum specimen must be obtained or when ventilation is compromised by secretions retained in the central airways. Suctioning is seldom needed more often than hourly. Blindly placed, a suction catheter usually reaches the lower trachea or right main bronchus and recovers sputum from more distal airways only if cough propels sputum forward. It may trigger laryngospasm, bronchospasm, and cardiac arrhythmias. Even if sterile, the catheter introduces large innocula of pharyngeal bacteria into the lower tract, and suction traumatizes respiratory mucosa (thereby injuring the mucociliary escalator). Suctioning may also induce hypoxemia, either by replacing oxygen with room air in the alveolar spaces or by causing microatelectasis, especially in patients removed from high levels of PEEP.

Proper technique emphasizes hygienic, but not sterile, precautions. "Pre-oxygenation" is accomplished by several deep inflations of 100% O_2 (via a manual resuscitation bag). Once the trachea is entered, the catheter is advanced 4-5 inches and then withdrawn as intermittent suction is applied for no longer than 5 seconds, total. Several "hyperinflations" of oxygen are given before resuming the usual ventilatory pattern.

OXYGEN THERAPY: GAS SOURCES

In most hospitals, both air and oxygen are available from two sources: wall lines pressurized at approximately 50 pounds per square inch (psi) and heavy metal cylinders that store compressed gas under approximately 2000 psi. Pressure-regulating valves reduce cylinder pressure to working levels, usually 50 psi. Flow meters adjusted to this working pressure govern the rate of gas delivery and can be attached directly to the wall source or to the regulating valve of the cylinder. Standard flow meters are calibrated to 15 liters/min but will allow delivery of much greater quantities of gas (approximately 50 liters/min) when the thumbscrew of the valve is turned wide open (flush or flood). All medical gases exiting directly from the source are dry and must be humidified to avoid dessication of upper respiratory tissues, except at very low rates of administration.

Cylinders of various medical gases are color coded: Air - silver or blue; O_2 - green or white; CO_2 - gray; Helium - brown.

Cylinder size is designated by alphabetical letters; E (4½" x 30"), G (8½" x 55"), and H (9" x 55") are used most frequently.

At a delivery rate of 2 liters/min a full E tank will last 5 hours and an H tank 57 hours. The duration of gas flow remaining at a given rate of use can be estimated for each cylinder size by the formula:

$$\text{Duration (in min)} = \frac{\text{gauge pressure (in psi) x cylinder factor}}{\text{flow rate (in l/min)}}$$

Cylinder factors are 0.28 for E, 2.41 for G, and 3.14 for H tanks.

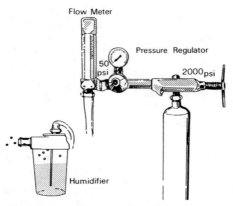

Figure 16.1. A gas delivery system: oxygen cylinder, pressure regulator, flow meter, and humidifier.

OXYGEN THERAPY: METHODS OF O_2 ADMINISTRATION

Sufficient supplemental oxygen should be administered to keep hemoglobin at least 85-90% saturated ($\approx$ 60 mmHg). Maintaining arterial oxygen tensions in excess of 70 mmHg can prove detrimental to patients with depressed ventilatory drives and is only necessary for protracted periods in unusual circumstances (e.g., severe and symptomatic anemia, ongoing myocardial or cerebral ischemia).

Nasal Cannulae (Prongs), Nasal and Transtracheal Catheters

Nasal prongs are perhaps the best choice for most applications requiring moderate oxygen supplementation. Continuous flow fills the nasopharynx and oropharynx with oxygen. These reservoirs empty into the lungs during each tidal breath, even when breath occurs through a widely open mouth. One of the two prongs can be taped flat (or cut off and the hole sealed) without a notable change in F_iO_2, allowing effective supplementation to continue despite the presence of an occlusive nasogastric tube, nasotracheal suction catheter, or bronchoscope in the other nostril. More importantly, nasal prongs allow the flow of oxygen to continue uninterrupted while eating or expectorating and during procedures involving the oropharynx (such as suctioning and orotracheal intubation). Prongs taped in place reliably delivery oxygen to patients who tend to remove face masks.

Rates of nasal oxygen administration vary from ½ to 6 liters per minute. At a fixed oxygen flow rate, the F_iO_2 achieved depends upon minute ventilation. Thus, a "low flow" rate of 2 liters per minute may correspond to a low or to a moderately high F_iO_2, depending on whether it is diluted with a large or small quantity of ambient air. For an average patient, 0.4 approximates the upper limit of F_iO_2 achievable by this method.

The jet of oxygen causes dryness of the nasal mucosa and pain in the paranasal sinuses at high flow rates. Oxygen must be humidified if given faster than 4 liters/min with two prongs or 2 liters/min with one prong. A nonpetroleum-based lubricating jelly applied to each nostril is a useful prophylactic measure against local irritation.

A nasal catheter is a single perforated plastic tube placed behind the soft palate. Somewhat more secure than nasal prongs, catheters deliver similar concentrations of oxygen. They are less popular than prongs because of greater irritation to nasal tissues, because location must be checked frequently, and because the catheter must be alternated between nostrils every 8 hours.

Delivery of oxygen via a soft, multiperforated <u>transtracheal</u> <u>catheter</u> has recently been introduced to clinical practice, with exciting initial results. The precise benefits, indications, and complications of this methodology are not well worked out at the present time. However, initial data indicate that rates of oxygen utilization are much lower than with nasal appliances and that patient acceptance and compliance for long-term use are encouraging.

Face Masks

Face masks can be used to provide higher oxygen concentrations than are available with open tents and nasal devices but are inherently uncomfortable and less stable than other methods delivering similar inspired fractions of oxygen. Masks must be removed when eating and expectorating, allowing the oxygen concentration to fall during these activities. Patients often discard them when agitated, dyspneic, or asleep.

There are five common types of face mask: simple, partial rebreathing, nonrebreathing, open tent, and Venturi. <u>Simple masks</u> have an oxygen inlet at the base and holes at the sides to allow exhalation. Because peak inspiratory flow rate usually exceeds the inflow rate of oxygen, room air is entrained around the mask and through the side holes. Hence, the F_iO_2 actually delivered depends not only upon the oxygen flow rate but also upon the patient's tidal volume and inspiratory flow pattern. In an "average" patient, the oxygen percentage delivered by a simple mask varies from approximately 35% at 6 liters/min to 55% at 10 liters/min. At low flow rates, CO_2 can collect in the mask, effectively adding dead space and increasing the work of breathing.

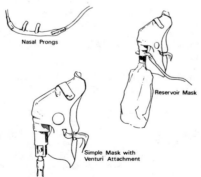

Nasal Prongs

Reservoir Mask

Simple Mask with
Venturi Attachment

<u>Figure 16.2.</u> Three methods of oxygen administration.

Partial-rebreather (reservoir) masks are used commonly but have few advantages over the simple mask. The structure is virtually identical to the simple mask, but oxygen flows continuously into a collapsible reservoir bag attached to the base. If the mask is well sealed, the patient draws from the bag when demand exceeds the constant line supply. Peak flows draw less air from the room and a higher F_iO_2 is achieved. Upon exhalation the first portion of exhaled (oxygen-rich) gas helps refill the reservoir, and the rest vents to atmosphere via the side ports. The reservoir must be kept filled; if the bag is allowed to collapse, the partial rebreather converts to a simple mask. Although these masks make more efficient use of oxygen, the highest F_iO_2 usually achievable with this device is approximately 0.65 at 10 liters of oxygen inflow.

Nonrebreather masks are identical to partial rebreather masks, except for two sets of one-way valves. One valve set is placed between the reservoir and the body of the mask so that exhaled gas must exit through the side ports or around the mask. The second valve set seals one or both side ports during inspiration so that nearly all inhaled gas is drawn from the oxygen reservoir. With a tight fitting mask, effective concentrations of 90-95% can be delivered. Oxygen inflow must be adjusted high enough to prevent collapse of the reservoir bag. Should collapse occur, oxygen delivery rate would be insufficient to meet minute ventilation requirements, causing the patient to struggle against the one-way valves to entrain additional room air. Masks without a safety release mechanism could conceivably allow a weak or restrained patient to suffocate. Hence, patients on nonrebreather masks must be kept under direct observation continuously.

Open face tents can be used to deliver either oxygen or mist. They allow the patient to communicate with personnel and expectorate easily but impede eating. The inspired oxygen fraction (F_iO_2) varies widely with the set flow rate, tent positioning, and minute ventilation. Inspired oxygen fractions cannot be boosted above 0.6 because of entrainment of ambient air. Open tents serve a useful purpose in patients who will not tolerate tight-fitting face masks or nasal cannulae.

With all of the methods of oxygen delivery discussed thus far, F_iO_2 can vary depending on the patient's breathing pattern. In certain clinical situations, such as decompensated COPD with CO_2 retention, more precise control may be desired. Venturi masks provide a concentration of oxygen no higher than that specified. Oxygen is directed into a jet, which entrains room air to flood the facial area with a gas mixture of fixed oxygen concentration. If the patient's peak inspiratory rate does not exceed the combined flow of the oxygen-air mixture, the F_iO_2 will be the nominal value, provided that the mask fits snugly. Venturi masks are available to deliver selected oxygen percentages varying from 24 to 50%. Some masks allow rapid switching of the delivered concentration by adjustment of a collar selector, which changes the entrainment ratio.

Endotracheal Tubes

Any inspired fraction of oxygen can be given when a cuffed endotracheal tube prevents access to room air. If the patient is not connected to a ventilator circuit, humidified gas is administered either by a T-piece adapter or a tracheostomy tent. If no "tail" (wide-bore tubing) is attached to the T-adapter, the concentration of oxygen delivered will be less than that in the afferent tubing because of dilution by room air. A length of tubing attached downstream from the endotracheal tube orifice provides an inspiratory reservoir to counteract this effect without adding to dead space. The length needed depends on the source flow rate and the patient's peak flow demand.

A tracheostomy mask is a small, open-domed hood that creates a tent-like area over the tracheostomy orifice. Some room air entrainment occurs, tending to reduce both humidity and F_iO_2. The latter can usually be overcome by increasing the oxygen fraction. The trach mask is less unwieldly than a T-piece and does not produce traction on the tube.

HUMIDITY AND HUMIDIFICATION

Normally, gas at the carinal level is fully humidified at a temperature approaching 37°C. The amount of water vapor in gas that remains in contact with a moist surface (and therefore is fully saturated) depends uniquely upon temperature. At a given temperature, water vapor exerts a fixed tension, independent of the total pressure of the mixture.

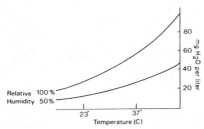

Figure 16.3. Effect of temperature on water vapor content of saturated gas. Because the capacity of gas for water increases dramatically with temperature, a substantial amount of water must be added as inspired gas is warmed to 37°C, even if the gas was fully saturated at room temperature (23°C).

During spontaneous normal breathing most of this water is supplied by the well-vascularized mucosa of the nasal and oral passages. At normal rates of breathing the nose is an efficient air conditioner, filtering out particles greater than 10 microns in size and completing the warming and humidifying process before gas enters the larynx. The mouth is somewhat less effective, especially at high minute ventilation. If humidification is not completed in the upper airway, water must be drawn from the tracheobronchial mucosa, causing dessication, impaired mucociliary clearance, and thickened sputum.

Unlike ambient air (which is, on average, 50% saturated), medical gases contain no water vapor, so that the entire amount must be supplied. Unhumidified gas can cause drying of the nasal and oral mucosa. Should the upper airway be bypassed, as by endotracheal intubation, drying of the sensitive lower tract occurs, with the attendant risk of infection and ventilatory impairment. The object of external humidification is to provide gas containing acceptable amounts of water vapor to the respiratory tract. Gas introduced at the tracheal level must be fully prewarmed and saturated. If the upper tract is not bypassed, humidity and temperature similar to those of ambient air suffice.

Without the upper airway bypassed, low flow rates of oxygen (e.g., up to 3 liters by nasal prongs) admix with sufficient ambient air to preclude the need for humidification, unless the ambient environment is exceptionally dry. External humidification is required with higher flow rates by prongs and with masks that deliver moderate to high oxygen concentrations.

Humidifiers are of several types: pass-over, bubble, jet, and heated units, in increasing order of efficiency. Pass-over units direct the gas stream tangentially over a water surface and serve well only at very low flow rates. Bubble (diffuser) humidifiers break the gas stream into bubbles under water, increasing the surface area for contact and rendering them useful for low to moderate flow applications. Relative humidity of the gas produced varies directly with flow rate. Jet nebulizers produce macroscopic water particles, which are carried by the gas stream. Depending upon the particular type of unit and the flow rate, water droplets may evaporate completely before reaching the patient, in which case these units act as true humidifiers. More often, particulate water is delivered, in addition to vapor.

Raising the temperature of a gas increases its capacity to hold water. Air fully saturated at room temperature needs additional moisture when warmed by inhalation. Prior heating is mandatory if adequate moisture is to be supplied through an endotracheal tube, unless particulate (aerosolized) water is also administered. The latter is relatively disadvantageous because particulate water increases the likelihood of innoculating the lower respiratory tract with bacteria. To avoid excessive mucosal hydration the temperature of the humidified gas mixture should not exceed 33-34°C. It should be noted that gas supersaturated at 37°C will form a mist as it contacts the cooler (23°C) room air, which is unable to hold as much moisture. Thus, a mist produced from the end of a T-piece or exiting from a mask does not necessarily imply that particulate water is being delivered. Rather, if mist is not seen, it implies that full humidification of warmed gas is not occurring.

AEROSOL THERAPY

Aerosols are suspensions of liquid (or solid) macroparticles in gas. Common therapeutic purposes of aerosol therapy are to deliver medication, to induce productive coughing, to decrease laryngeal edema, and to add water to the tracheobronchial tree to aid sputum clearance. Inhalation is a particularly attractive way to deliver medication because high topical concentrations result in favorable therapeutic ratios.

Aerosols are characterized by the size and homogeneity of the particles. The larger the size of the particle, the more proximally it deposits in the airway. Turbulent flow produced by forceful breathing or airways obstruction increases the fraction of particles deposited centrally, regardless of size. Thus, aerosols distribute poorly in badly obstructed patients because they do not reach distal airways.

Bronchodilator Aerosols

Only a small fraction of the prescribed dose of aerosolized medication actually deposits within the airway, due to deposition in the nebulizing device, the oropharynx, ventilator tubing, etc. To maximize efficiency, inhalation should be deep, slow, and held for 2-3 seconds at total lung capacity. To maximize the percentage of drug reaching the patient, the dose should be delivered in at least 2 ml of diluent. A given dose of bronchodilator should be delivered by multiple breaths over a 5-15 minute period in order to allow bronchodilatation resulting from initial inhalations to assist the distal deposition of later inhalations. Since a large percentage of the dose deposits in the oropharynx, it is wise to have the patient rinse the pharynx with water and expectorate after administration of an absorbable medication.

Other Medicinal Aerosols

Certain irritating medications may produce bronchospasm in susceptible patients. Mucolytic drugs are notable in this regard and for this reason should be mixed with, or preceded by, a bronchodilator. The clinical use of steroid aerosols and cromolyn are discussed elsewhere (see p. 182). To date, antibiotic aerosols have no well-accepted clinical indication.

Delivery of Medication

Many types of nebulizer are available for medication delivery; the choice should reflect the intended purpose.

(1) An atomizer produces a range of very large particles (10-30 microns) and is ideal for topical delivery of medication to the larynx, as when preparing to intubate the trachea.

(2) Small-volume jet nebulizers produce an aerosol of particles 2-8 microns in diameter. Various forms of such nebulizers can be attached to ventilators or IPPB machines, or used independently, with gas supplied by a compressor or wall source. Modes employing positive pressure (IPPB) are no more effective than deep spontaneous inhalations unless the patient is too weak to deep-breathe.

(3) Metered-dose nebulizers (canister "inhalers") use a compressed-gas propellent to expel a measured puff of medication when actuated. Their compact portable size and the requirement for patient coordination suits them best for outpatient use. Spacing chambers suspend the dose, rendering the timing of canister activation less critical.

(4) Ultrasonic nebulizers use high-frequency vibrations to impart enough energy to aerosolize the fluid and are capable of delivering a high volume (to 6 ml/min) of uniform, small (less than 5 microns) particles that reach deeply into the tracheobronchial tree. Few patients can tolerate continuous ultrasonic therapy without coughing or sensing dyspnea. (Many patients with hyperreactive airways experience bronchospasm.) Hence, ultrasonics are best used intermittently for sputum induction or medication delivery. Bland aerosol administration using this unit should only be done for brief periods as part of a respiratory therapy treatment for patients with thickened secretions.

Bland (Water) Aerosols

Very few data document benefit from adding water topically to the tracheobronchial tree, above that needed for adequate humidification. Some evidence suggests that only the surface layers of preformed sputum take up water, causing swelling but little change in viscosity. The lubricated surface layers may allow sputum to shear more easily from airway walls, allowing expectoration.   However, secretions that nearly plug small airways may become occlusive when hydrated. Large-volume aerosols may cause massive outpouring of tracheobronchial secretions and overcome the clearance capacity of a debilitated patient. Furthermore, unlike vapor, water droplets may carry bacteria into the lung. Finally, high volumes of small particles, especially of distilled water or hypertonic saline, may cause sufficient irritation to trigger coughing and bronchospasm. (An inhaled bronchodilator should be delivered immediately before or concomitantly with high-volume bland aerosols.)

SUGGESTED READINGS

1.   Christopher KL, et al.   Transtracheal oxygen therapy for refractory hypoxemia. JAMA 1986;256:494-97.

2.   Helmholz HF Jr, Burton GG.   Applied humidity and aerosol therapy (Chapter 17). In: Burton GG, Hodgkin JE, eds. Respiratory Care. A Guide to Clinical Practice. Philadelphia: JB Lippincott, 1984:379-84.

3.   McPherson SP. Respiratory Therapy Equipment, 3rd ed. St. Louis: CV Mosby, 1985.

4.   Shapiro BA, Harrison RA, Trout CA. Clinical Application of Respiratory Care. Chicago: Yearbook Medical Publishers, 1985.

5.   Spearman CB, Sheldon RL. Egan's Fundamentals of Respiratory Therapy. St. Louis: CV Mosby, 1982.

Chapter 17

Bronchoscopy

Choice of Instrument

Bronchoscopy can be accomplished with a thin, flexible, fiberoptic instrument or with a large-diameter rigid tube and telescopes. The flexible instrument has a tip that can be directed into all the major and segmental bronchi, making it well suited for diagnostic work. Several calibers are available for use in pediatric and adult patients. It can be inserted either transnasally or through an oral endotracheal tube of appropriate diameter (8.5 mm or larger for the standard 5-mm bronchoscope). During mechanical ventilation, the fiberscope can be passed through the lumen of a large oral tube or alongside the cuff of a smaller airway.

The rigid instrument offers inspection confined to the central airways but can secure large biopsies within that limited range and allows better visualization, suctioning, and control of vigorously bleeding central lesions.

Diagnostic Uses

Fiberoptic bronchoscopy can be used to inspect the larynx and lower airway to the subsegmental level and to biopsy lesions within that range under direct vision. Nonvisualized peripheral lesions often can be biopsied under fluoroscopic guidance using small forceps and brushes. A hollow (Wang) needle can be passed through the wall of the tracheal or main bronchus to probe mediastinal nodes and submucosal tumors. This technique is also helpful for diagnosis of friable and highly vascular endobronchial lesions.

The fiberoptic bronchoscope cannot, however, direct a sampling instrument with equal facility into all areas of the lung. The biopsy forceps fails to make the sharply angled turns needed to reliably follow the appropriate bronchus beyond the subsegmental level, because the tip of the forceps itself is not maneuverable. Hence, lesions in certain locations are inaccessible, especially if small. This is particularly true for segments sharply angulated from the main bronchi, such as the apical segments of the upper lobes and the superior segments of the lower lobes. Other lesions (e.g., metastases) do not communicate directly with a bronchus at all. Some apparently "hilar" tumors originate in small airways but appear to overlie central bronchi on chest radiographs.

Parenchymal biopsy (transbronchial biopsy, TBB) can be performed safely in patients with intact or compromised immune defenses, provided that the risk of bleeding is acceptable. Although the tissue fragments obtained are small, they can be used to establish diagnoses of sarcoidosis, tuberculosis, neoplasia, certain infiltrative diseases, and infection due to pneumocystis or fungi. A diagnosis of vasculitis cannot generally be made because sizable vessels are not obtained. Furthermore, many parenchymal diseases are patchy, with different stages of the process present in different areas. Hence, the samples recovered may not represent the entire process. If TBB is nondiagnostic, open biopsy should be considered.

Passing the fiberscope through the oropharynx contaminates the lower airway, rendering bacterial cultures invalid. However, a sheathed (protected) catheter technique is available with which uncontaminated parenchymal cultures can be obtained.

As an aid to diagnosis of distal endobronchial and parenchymal disease, segmental lavage can be done to obtain cells for differential counting, cytology, and microbiologic processing. With this technique, the scope is wedged into a lobar or segmental bronchus and large aliquots of sterile saline solution (e.g., 50 ml x 4) are gently instilled and withdrawn. Lavage appears to be an especially effective technique when attempting to diagnose infections in patients with AIDS and other immune-compromised hosts. Washings consistent with pneumocystis, atypical mycobacteriosis, cytomegalovirus, and fungal pathogens can often be recovered when biopsies are unrevealing or contraindicated by bleeding tendency or bullous lung disease. Selective bronchography is also feasible.

Rigid bronchoscopy is a viable alternative when hemoptysis is vigorous and when the pieces of a centrally located tumor recovered with the fiberoptic instrument are too small to be interpreted with confidence.

Therapeutic Uses

Intubation of the trachea over the fiberoptic instrument can be done easily, even in otherwise difficult cases. It can also facilitate selective or double lumen intubation. However, other therapeutic uses of the fiberoptic instrument are somewhat limited by its narrow channel and the tendency of blood and secretions to cloud the image. Small foreign objects can be extracted with the forceps or with special snares and baskets. Accumulated secretions unresponsive to chest physiotherapy are often loosened and dislodged. Refractory lobar atelectasis may respond to this approach. Abscess cavities can be probed in an attempt to establish drainage in difficult cases, but extreme care must be taken to prevent aspiration of infected material. A thin balloon catheter can be directed with a fiberscope and inflated to stanch a parenchymal hemorrhage (see p. 223). In recent years fiberoptic and laser technologies have been linked to produce a cauterizing instrument capable of endobronchial oblative surgery. Tissue excision of occlusive lesions and photocoagulation within the central airway are two important applications of this technique.

The rigid instrument is better suited for many therapeutic purposes. It is especially useful when extracting large foreign objects and when performing limited tamponade or packing of the bronchus. Thick or copious large airway secretions can be aspirated easily through its large channel. During massive hemoptysis the ventilating bronchoscope can be inserted into the nonbleeding side to prevent asphyxia.

Complications

Infection

Several factors contribute to the risk of infection. Because the bronchoscope must pass the pharynx, it contaminates the lower airway passages with large inoculum of bacteria. Topical anesthesia of the pharynx and tracheobronchial tree blunts the reflexes that protect against aspiration. Furthermore, lidocaine and atropine slow the mucociliary escalator. A low-grade fever that usually abates spontaneously (without antibiotics) is common 12-24 hours following bronchoscopy, presumably due to subclinical pneumonitis. Extensive lavage tends to increase the incidence of pyrexia. Occasionally, overt pneumonia develops, especially if the instrument was passed beyond an obstructed airway or through a region of mucopurulent secretions.

Aspiration

Sedation and local anesthesia impair the protective laryngeal reflexes and swallowing for several hours. In addition, the large doses of lidocaine required to control coughing often cause confusion and lethargy in the elderly. Hence, patients should be kept NPO for several hours and only allowed to ingest food after water is swallowed without difficulty. The patient remains at risk for massive aspiration of food, liquids, and gastric contents for several hours after bronchoscopy. When the stimulation of the procedure ceases, an apparently alert patient may become obtunded, compounding the hazard. Patients must be assessed carefully for any sign of depressed mental status.

If a lung abscess has been probed, the airway may flood with purulent material that cannot be eliminated by a depressed cough. Life-threatening pneumonia may result. In such cases, the affected lung should be placed in a dependent position and the patient kept for several hours under continued observation.

Bronchospasm and Airway Obstruction

Manipulation of the airway stimulates irritant receptors, causing bronchospasm in many patients with asthma or COPD. In this setting, anticholinergic bronchodilators, such as atropine, are particularly effective. Mucosal edema adds to the degree of obstruction.

Hypoxemia

In patients with abnormal lungs, hypoxemia related to bronchoscopy may continue for 6-12 hours postprocedure, especially if lavage was extensive. If hypoxemia is suspected, supplemental oxygen should be continued during that period.

Pneumothorax

If transbronchial biopsies are taken from sites adjacent to the visceral pleura (such as near an interlobar fissure), pneumothorax may result. Rarely, a brush extended too peripherally or vigorous hard coughing during the procedure can cause the same problem. The pneumothorax is usually minor, not requiring a chest tube. However, the leak can develop slowly over several hours, so that the postbiopsy chest film should be delayed at least 90 minutes if the patient remains asymptomatic. During mechanical ventilation, parenchymal biopsy can cause a tension pneumothorax. Pneumothorax may also result during mechanical ventilation when the fiberscope is passed through an endotracheal tube of inadequate dimension. In this setting, transient airway obstruction can cause dangerous levels of parenchymal pressure to develop, an "auto-PEEP" effect, with attendant risks of hypotension and barotrauma.

Bleeding

Minor hemoptysis (sputum streaking) that persists for 12-48 hours after the procedure is common after biopsy. Major hemorrhage is rare, except in poorly selected patients with clotting abnormalities. Prebiospy data must include a platelet count, coagulation studies, and BUN. Aspirin should be withheld for at least 3 days before the procedure. Occasionally, bronchoscopy must be done on a patient whose platelet count is less than $50,000/mm^3$ or whose coagulation status is impaired. Under these conditions biopsy is hazardous and should be attempted only if clearly necessary and with platelet or clotting factor support.

Pulmonary hypertension is a strong risk factor for bleeding from parenchymal, but not bronchial, biopsies. Bronchial adenomas are reported to bleed excessively when biopsied, but this admonition may be overemphasized.

SUGGESTED READINGS

1. Anderson HA, Faber LP, eds. Diagnostic and therapeutic applications of the bronchoscope (Suppl). Chest 1978;73:685-778.

2. Dreisen RB, et al. Flexible fiberoptic bronchoscopy in the teaching hospital. Yield and complications. Chest 1978;74:144-49.

3. Fulkerson WJ. Fiberoptic bronchoscopy. N. Engl. J. Med. 1984;311:511-15.

4. Lindholm CE, et al. Cardiorespiratory effects of flexible fiberoptic bronchoscopy in critically ill patients. Chest 1978;74:362-68.

5. Sackner MA. Bronchofiberscopy - State of the Art. Am. Rev. Respir. Dis. 1975;111:62-88.

6. Stover DE, et al. Diagnosis of pulmonary disease in acquired immune deficiency syndrome. Am. Rev. Respir. Dis. 1984;130:659-62.

7. Stradling P. Diagnostic Bronchoscopy, 3rd ed. London: Churchill Livingstone, 1986.

8. Suratt PM, Smiddy JF, Graber B. Deaths and complications associated with fiberoptic bronchoscopy. Chest 1976;69:747-51.

9. Zavala DC. Flexible Fiberoptic Bronchoscopy. Iowa City: University of Iowa Press, 1978.

Chapter 18

Nonbronchoscopic Lung Biopsy and Mediastinoscopy

NONBRONCHOSCOPIC LUNG BIOPSY

Lung tissue may be sampled by four common techniques: 1) transthoracic needle aspiration, 2) transthoracic cutting needle biopsy, 3) transbronchial biopsy, and 4) open thoracotomy. Tissue may be required to determine the etiology of an acute infection, to determine the nature of a chronic infiltrative process, or to determine the composition of a parenchymal mass or nodule.

Aspiration Needle Biopsy

Using fluoroscopic or CT-scan guidance, a long thin needle is inserted through the chest wall into the parenchyma. In practiced hands, even lesions close to the great vessels of the hilum may be approached safely. Since only an aspirate of tissue fluid is obtained, the specimen is suitable for cytology, stain, and culture, but not histopathologic analysis. Appropriate applications are to determine the benign or malignant nature of a solitary pulmonary nodule, to determine the etiology of acute pneumonitis, and to sample the contents of an intraparenchymal cyst or abscess. Lesions of greater than 1.5 cm diameter can usually be sampled. Needle aspiration cannot usually diagnose a benign lesion. However, if a malignant nodule is entered, the chances of recovering positive cytology are approximately 80%. Attempting a needle aspirate of a lung lesion seems rational when a patient is reluctant to go to surgery without proof of malignancy or when the physician is inclined to follow the radiographic appearance of a nodule of uncertain age.

Pneumothorax is the major complication, occurring in approximately 25-30% of cases. Chest tube drainage will be necessary in only one-third of these. Minor hemoptysis is common but significant hemorrhage is rare. Seeding of the needle tract or pleura with tumor cells is not a problem. Unless pleural symphysis is certain, needles of any kind should not be inserted into patients with only one functional lung or into obviously bullous tissue.

Cutting Needle Biopsy

Many types of cutting needles have been devised, all providing macroscopic tissue for histologic examination. With the possible exception of the Nordenstrom needle (which provides very small tissue fragments), cutting needle biopsy dramatically increases the risk of serious bleeding and pneumothorax, with only marginally improved yield over aspiration technique. Cutting needle biopsy should be reserved for lesions adherent to the chest wall, such as superior sulcus (Pancoast) tumors, or for very peripheral lesions with obvious pleural symphysis. Serious hemorrhage can result from deep parenchymal biopsy because of the large thin-walled vessels present centrally.

Transbronchial Biopsy (TBB) vs. Needle Biopsy

TBB is discussed under Bronchoscopy (see p. 103). A decision must often be made whether to approach a lesion endobronchially or percutaneously. If the lesion can be successfully entered, the sample obtained bronchoscopically is more likely to establish the diagnosis. By providing tissue for histology, precise tumor typing and confirmation of benign diagnoses can be accomplished. Furthermore, TBB has a lower associated incidence of pneumothorax (10%) and provides the opportunity to inspect the endobronchial tree for associated pathology.

The likelihood of obtaining tissue from a small or peripheral nodule, however, is considerably higher for needle than for bronchoscopic biopsy, especially if the nodule is located in an area poorly accessible by TBB. Infiltrative lesions are best approached bronchoscopically because, except for routine bacterial pneumonia, tissue is usually required to establish a diganosis. Transbronchial biopsy is also the method of choice when attempting to secure tissue to diagnose sarcoidosis; noncaseating granulomas can be recovered in 65% of radiographic stage I and 85% of stage II patients.

Open Biopsy

Open lung biopsy provides a large piece of tissue and hence is subject to less sampling error than other methods when investigating patchy diffuse infiltrates. Despite the need for thoracotomy, the procedure is quite well tolerated, even by seriously ill patients. Open biopsy allows better hemostasis and is therefore preferred for diagnosis of infiltrative disease in patients with clotting abnormalities.

Open biopsy is logically the first procedure to be done in many cases of suspicious nodules in operable patients because needle aspiration and transbronchial biopsy often fail to prove benign diagnoses, whereas a diagnosis of malignancy mandates removal. Malignant nodules can be removed in their entirety at the time of diagnosis. However, prior needle aspiration or bronchoscopy is indicated when there is an inclination to wait and watch carefully unless malignancy is proven (e.g., a contraindication to surgery or a strong suspicion of benign disease). Because most small cell cancers should be treated by chemotherapy rather than by surgery, this provides another rationale for attempts at nonoperative diagnosis.

In cases of pneumonia in <u>immune-compromised hosts,</u> a precise diagnosis can eventually be made in approximately 60% of cases. Bronchial brushing, lavage, and transbronchial biopsy can potentially diagnose about 60% of these without need for thoracotomy. However, there are several major concerns with bronchoscopic technique in this setting:

1) Bleeding - Many of these patients are thrombocytopenic. The risk of bleeding is not entirely obviated by platelet transfusions. Open biopsy is safer.

2) Sampling error - Small TBB pieces may miss the responsible pathogen or recover only one of several organisms. Furthermore, noninfectious processes (radiation pneumonitis, graft-versus-host disease, etc.) cannot be diagnosed confidently from such limited tissue.

3) Impaired oxygenation - Very high oxygen fractions cannot be maintained during bronchoscopy. Furthermore, TBB cannot be performed safely in patients receiving mechanical ventilation.

4) Delayed treatment of a life-threatening process - Complete processing of specimens requires hours to days in most hospitals. If bronchoscopy does not make the diagnosis, appropriate treatment may be delayed.

5) Introduction of oral pathogens into the lower tract.

As a general strategy, a full or modified fiberoptic bronchoscopic procedure should be considered as the first step for all but the most seriously ill or rapidly deteriorating patients. Open biopsy is appropriate if the bronchoscopy is unrevealing or if the severity or rate of progression requires immediate diagnosis. Empiric treatment with broad spectrum coverage against bacterial, fungal, and parasitic pathogens without biopsy confirmation is an alternative strategy but exposes the patient to the costs and hazards of prolonged, nondescript drug therapy.

MEDIASTINOSCOPY

Indications

Mediastinoscopy affords access to the nodes that drain the lungs without requiring thoracotomy. The three major indications for this procedure are 1) to assess operability of known bronchogenic carcinoma, 2) to obtain lymphoid tissue in order to establish the diagnosis of granulomatous disease, and 3) to investigate mediastinal masses. When positive for carcinoma, subcarinal transbronchial (Wang) needle aspiration can obviate the need for further mediastinal investigation, especially when the computerized tomographic (CT) scan demonstrates a mass lesion or node greater in diameter than 1.5 cm. Patients under consideration for curative resection of a lung tumor should undergo a staging workup of the mediastinum that includes a CT, followed by a mediastinoscopic procedure, if positive. It should be emphasized that CT scans are not uniformly sensitive or specific, and unexpected results are found with surprising frequency.

Method

Although some surgeons mediastinoscope all patients with potentially operable carcinoma, most use a selective approach. Cell type and tumor location influence mediastinoscopic yield. Cases having a sufficiently high incidence of positive findings to warrant the procedure are those with 1) involvement of the central bronchi, 2) radiograph or CT scan suspicious for involvement of the mediastinum, 3) adenocarcinoma or undifferentiated cell type, 4) constitutional symptoms, and 5) peripheral masses greater than 2.0 cm in diameter.

Mediastinal inspection is usually performed through a neck incision made at the suprasternal notch. The space between the trachea and the pretracheal fascia can be followed to the carinal bifurcation and for a variable distance along each main bronchus. Pretracheal, subcarinal, and some hilar nodes can be sampled from the superior and posterior-middle mediastinum. Examination along the left paratracheal region and main bronchus is more difficult than on the right side because the aortic arch and pulmonary artery impede progress. Furthermore, left-sided lesions often metastasize first to the subaortic nodes, which cannot be reached by this route.

Surgical exploration of the anterior mediastinum (anterior mediastinotomy) appears to be a better approach when the lesion lies in the left lung or low on either side or when hilar nodes are radiographically involved beyond the reach of the mediastinoscope. In this procedure, the instrument is inserted into the anterior mediastinum through a <u>parasternal incision</u> made by removing the 2nd or 3rd costal cartilages. (Although associated with higher morbidity, some surgeons prefer to perform a "minithoracotomy" instead of anterior mediastinoscopy, opening the mediastinum more widely to direct vision and biopsy. Using this approach, the pleura can also be incised and a lung biopsy taken.)

Complications

With care and practice, complications are infrequent. However, severe hemorrhage (biopsy or tear of great vessels), pneumothorax, mediastinitis, and left recurrent laryngeal nerve injury can occur. Superior vena caval syndrome contraindicates mediastinoscopy because of bleeding and edema. Mediastinal fibrosis induced by granulomatous infection, radiotherapy, or a previous mediastinoscopy can render the technique impossible.

Mediastinoscopy is falsely negative in 10-15% of cases. Occasionally, grossly normal nodes are recovered that demonstrate involvement when sectioned carefully. For this reason, "double setup" procedures, in which mediastinoscopy and (if negative) thoracotomy are performed during the same anesthesia, are hazardous. However, if ipsilateral to the lesion and low in the mediastinum, most surgeons do not consider intranodal squamous cancer to contraindicate resection.

SUGGESTED READINGS

1. Hashim SW, Baue AE, Geha AS. The role of mediastinoscopy and mediastinotomy in lung cancer. <u>Clin. Chest Med.</u> 1982;3:353-59.

2. Loke J, Matthay RA, Ikeda S. Techniques for diagnosing lung cancer - A critical review. <u>Clin. Chest Med.</u> 1982;3:321-29.

3. Poe RH, Tobin RE. Sensitivity and specificity of needle biopsy in lung malignancy. <u>Am. Rev. Respir. Dis.</u> 1980;122:725-29.

4. Sagel SS, et al. Percutaneous transthoracic aspiration needle biopsy. <u>Ann. Thorac. Surg.</u> 1978;26:399-405.

5. Wallace JM, Deutsch AL. Flexible fiberoptic bronchoscopy and percutaneous needle lung aspiration for evaluating the solitary pulmonary nodule. <u>Chest</u> 1982;81:665-71.

6. Winston A, Schnurer LB. The value of mediastinoscopy - experience of 374 cases. <u>J. Otolaryngol.</u> 1978;7:103-09.

Chapter 19

The Chest Radiograph

TECHNICAL CONSIDERATIONS

Awareness of the limitations of radiographic technique helps to avoid misinterpretation. Films can be taken with the beam traversing the patient in posteroanterior (PA) or anteroposterior (AP) projections. Standard films are usually taken PA, while portable films are taken AP. With either, structures closest to the film are both sharper and less magnified than structures closer to the source. Similar considerations apply to lateral views. Hence, it is wise to request the lateral view that places the pathology closest to the film. (If unspecified, most departments take the left lateral view.)

Portable (AP) films magnify the heart and anterior mediastinum - an effect accentuated by the increased divergence of the x-ray beam caused by closer placement of the source to the film (3-4½ feet for AP vs. 6 feet for PA films). The kilovoltage chosen for AP portable films can emphasize rib and calcium contrast but "wash out" the lung parenchyma. Furthermore, the degree of penetration is difficult to control.

The patient is often neither supine nor upright when filmed. Hence, normal structures may apparently enlarge, air-fluid levels change, and ordinary silhouettes disappear, solely because of changing perspective. Lordosis causes apparent widening of the heart and mediastinum, as does rotation about the vertical axis. Unfortunately, the angle of inclination of "semiupright" films frequently changes and tilting the beam cannot compensate exactly. Many seriously ill patients cannot suspend inspiration. The result is a "breathing film," in which lung structures and diaphragms are blurred or an "exhalation film" that accentuates infiltrates, interstitial structures such as vessels, and pleural air or fluid. Changes in the phase of mechanical ventilation, in the tidal volume setting, or in the level of end-expiratory pressure can produce striking film-to-film variation.

SPECIAL VIEWS AND METHODS

Supine

Lung volume decreases in the supine position, highlighting infiltrates and interstitial structures. Venous return to the heart increases and azygous vein and pulmonary vessels distend. (A comparison of supine and upright films can be used to distinguish an azygous vein from an azygous node.) Blood flow redistributes to produce balanced perfusion to the upper and lower lobes. The images of the heart and mediastinal structures also enlarge because of an actual increase in distending pressures, as well as apparent widening caused by the rise of the diaphragms. Fluid and air migrate to dependent and non-dependent regions, respectively, so that sizable pleural effusions may appear only as a unilateral ground-glass haze over the affected hemithorax or a minor indentation laterally at entrance to a fissure, while small pneumothoraces and air-fluid levels within cavities disappear. Air migrates to the most superior regions. Two indications of pneumothorax on a supine film are the "deep sulcus" sign, in which the costophrenic angle or phrenomediastinal junctions are sharply and deeply outlined by air, and unusual hyperlucency superimposed on the liver shadow, caused by air in the anterior phrenocostal recess.

Expiration

A film taken unintentionally in expiration may give the misleading appearance of basilar infiltrates, increased heart size, and congested vessels. Inspiration/expiration films may be ordered deliberately to accentuate a pneumothorax. (A fixed amount of pleural air occupies a greater fraction of the thoracic volume during expiration.) Unilateral diaphragmatic paralysis and unilateral obstruction of a major bronchus are also demonstrated easily by this technique.

Lordotic

Disease in the posterior region of the apex and in the middle lobe is sometimes brought into better view with a lordotic film. Apical disease located anteriorly is often visualized best with a reverse lordotic view.

Obliques

Shadows of small lesions at the periphery of the lung can often be defined and separated from overlying shadows by filming at an oblique angle, especially when confusion regarding the lung or bony origin of a density is in question. Furthermore, lesions poorly seen on a lateral film can often be located with these views. Since ribs usually fracture in the anterior or posterior axillary lines, obliques are routinely used to define them.

Lateral Decubitus

Lateral decubitus filming with the beam centered over the region of interest allows detection of small amounts of fluid or air in the dependent or uppermost pleural space, respectively. This view also determines the size and mobility of a known collection of fluid (or air) and its accessibility to a sampling needle or tube. (A collection greater than 1 cm depth can usually be tapped.) Lung otherwise obscured by fluid may be uncovered by a decubitus view placing the involved lung uppermost. Thus, bilateral decubitus films may be useful even though only one pleural space contains fluid. Lateral decubitus films can be useful when assessing the mobility of mediastinal or pleural masses or of solids and fluids within cavities.

Because the uppermost lung is subjected to a moderately high distending pressure, the lateral decubitus position may permit a good "inspiration" film of that lung in an otherwise uncooperative patient.

High Penetration (Bucky) Films

If penetration is a problem, combining a high-energy beam with a moving grid (to reduce scatter) may be advantageous. Bucky films are valuable for patients with obesity, dense pleural or pulmonary opacities, lesions with calcium, or abnormalities obscured by heart and diaphragm. These views demonstrate air bronchograms and vessels in densely infiltrated areas clearly but may "burn out" minor infiltrates.

Valsalva and Müller Maneuvers

By changing intrathoracic pressure and venous return, the Valsalva and its obverse, the Müller maneuver, cause pulmonary vascular structures to shrink and distend, respectively. They are useful primarily when attempting to distinguish a vessel from a node or an A-V malformation from a solid lesion.

Barium Swallow

Apart from esophageal and stomach disease, a barium swallow can demonstrate enlarged retromediastinal nodes, outline a posterior intrathoracic mass, verify a ruptured or herniated diaphragm, or demonstrate impaired swallowing and aspiration.

Diagnostic Pneumothorax and Pneumoperitoneum

Placing a small quantity of air in the pleural space can distinguish a peripheral lung mass from a pleural lesion, outline a mesothelioma, or determine whether a parenchymal process extends to the chest wall. Associated complications are minimal when a blunt needle is used by experienced personnel. Pneumoperitoneum outlines the undersurface of the intact hemidiaphragm, allowing the depth of the thoracic cavity to be gauged.

INTERPRETATION

Checks Before Reading the Film

Written information - Note the name, date, time, and notations made by the technician (expiration, decubitus, etc.).

Position - Determine whether the film was taken supine, semiupright, or erect.

Alignment - Make note of whether the film was taken lordotic, kyphotic, or rotated laterally. (The distance between the heads of the clavicles should be split evenly by the dorsal spinous processes.)

Penetration - The intervertebral spaces should be just barely visible through the heart shadow. Films that are overpenetrated can sometimes be made more useful by "bright-lighting" them.

Systematic Review

There is a natural tendency to concentrate attention on obvious pathology. Many important but subtle findings will be missed unless adherence to a system forces review of all structures and areas. It does not matter what order is chosen, so long as lines and tubes, bones, soft tissues, pleural spaces, mediastinum, cardiovascular structures, lungs, and infradiaphragmatic areas are all scrutinized. Like physical examination, the review should be a "thinking" exercise, with attention keyed toward looking for the specific possible findings suggested by the clinical problem or other radiographic abnormalities.

Because perception of subtle findings improves as a film is viewed from different angles and distances, expert film readers "prowl" somewhat, stepping backward to gain better perspective, viewing the film at an angle to look for air bronchograms, faint nodules, etc. Radiographs are best viewed against moderately strong, even illumination. Surrounding panels should be extinguished and room lights should be dim. Definition of overpenetrated (dark) films often improves under bright focal lighting. Each area of the ribs and lung parenchyma should be compared with its contralateral counterpart.

Certain checks should be made routinely. Normally the hilum is higher and the hemidiaphragm lower on the left side, except in some elderly patients. The right hemidiaphragm should be sharply outlined, as should the left hemidiaphragm lateral to the cardiac apex. Any apparent lesion should be localized both on AP and lateral or oblique projections to fix its position within the thorax. Whenever an endotracheal tube is in place, its tip should be well cephalad of the carina, which normally overlies the level of the 5th-6th vertebral body. The entire anatomic course of all intravascular, gastrointestional catheters should be traced from their sites of insertion.

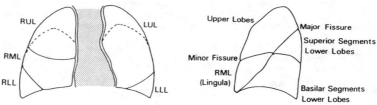

Figure 19.1. Radiographic lobar anatomy.

Specific Findings

Silhouette Sign

Loss of a normal border between structures of different radiodensity or appearance of a normally invisible outline can be an invaluable clue to the presence of infiltrates, fluid, or air. Occasionally, however, "false positives" occur (as on a poorly penetrated or badly aligned film or in the presence of anatomic variants of chest wall and diaphragm).

Air Bronchogram

When present, an air bronchogram is pathognomonic of consolidation or atelectasis. However, poorly penetrated films often fail to demonstrate them. By denoting an air-containing bronchus surrounded by collapsed or consolidated tissue, air visible within the bronchus means that secretions are able to exit from the region and that pneumonia or atelectasis is unlikely to persist solely because of proximal airway obstruction. Conversely, the absence of an air-bronchogram with an apparently routine lobar pneumonia should suggest the possibility of a central tumor.

Fissures and Septae

Normal fissures and septae frequently are not seen on rotated or under-penetrated films. Conversely, azygous and right medial basal fissures occasionally cause confusion, especially when their accessory segments are infiltrated, simulating mass lesions. Often, fissures are incompletely formed, accounting for collateral ventilation despite main airway blockage.

Lobar Collapse

In the absence of collateral ventilation, air distal to an obstruction usually reabsorbs in 4-24 hours (faster if the patient is on supplemental oxygen). If the central bronchus remains open, an air bronchogram may be seen despite parenchymal atelectasis, indicating that disordered regional mechanics are responsible for collapse. Primary signs of acute collapse include mediastinal shift (whole lung and lower lobe collapse), tracheal deviation (whole lung collapse), upward displacement of the hilum (upper lobe collapse), downward hilar displacement (lower lobe collapse), and shift of fissures (any segment). Narrowing of costal interspaces and compensatory hyperaeration of adjacent tissue are other key findings of massive atelectasis.

Hilar Node Enlargement

Unilateral hilar node enlargement usually signifies neoplasia, primary tuberculosis, sarcoidosis (8% of cases), or primary fungal infection. Bilateral hilar node enlargement usually results from sarcoidosis or lymphoma but can be simulated by an expiration film or pulmonary hypertension.

Uncurving Lines

With a few obvious exceptions, straight lines of substantial length are not normally found in the chest. A vertical line may indicate pneumothorax, artifact, or skin fold. Unlike the pleural line of pneumothorax, skin folds may extend beyond the rib margins, have only one definable edge, and fade gradually into the surrounding tissue, without abrupt termination. Perfectly horizontal lines indicate an air-fluid interface in the lung (abscess, cyst) or pleural space (hydropneumothorax, empyema). Distinction between intra- and extraparenchymal fluid collections can usually be made by their geometric appearance. Abscesses tend to have a similar diameter in both PA and lateral projections and often do not extend to the chest wall. The fluid line of an empyema tends to be disproportionately lengthy in one projection and always extends to the thoracic limit in one view or another.

Interstitial vs. Alveolar Infiltrates

Very few processes are confined exclusively to air spaces or to interstitium. Signs of alveolar filling include segmental distribution, coalescence, fluffy margins, air bronchograms, rosette patterns, and silhouetting of normal structures. If none are present, a diffuse infiltrate is likely to be largely interstitial. Far-advanced interstitial processes can produce many of these "alveolar" signs. Earlier interstitial infiltrates tend to follow the distribution of the pulmonary vasculature. Honeycombing is a reliable sign of an advanced interstitial process.

Any diffuse interstitial process will appear more radiodense at the bases than at the apices, in part because there is more tissue to penetrate. Alveoli are also smaller at the bases, so that the ratio of aerated volume to tissue volume declines near the diaphragm.

Terminology for Interstitial Infiltrates

Reticular: short linear and curved densities, irregularly distributed

Nodular: discrete rounded small densities of varying sizes, occasionally confluent

Miliary: many small regular densities, of more or less uniform size

Kerley's lines: Kerley's lines signify thickened septae or congested lymphatics and are usually seen in chronic left heart failure or lymphangitic carcinoma. True Kerley lines are seldom if ever seen in acute congestion or volume overload.

A lines: long linear shadows in the upper lobes, oriented perpendicularly to the pleura

B lines: short, linear horizontal shadows near the costophrenic angles of lower lobes

C lines: spiderweb network anywhere in the lungs

Pulmonary Edema

Pulmonary edema may result from increased vascular permeability or increased hydrostatic pressure. Recent work strongly suggests that the adult respiratory distress syndrome (ARDS), volume overload, and cardiogenic etiologies may produce distinct radiographic findings. In making a separation three primary considerations are important: the width of the vascular pedicle, the pulmonary blood flow distribution, and the pattern of parenchymal infiltration (lung edema).

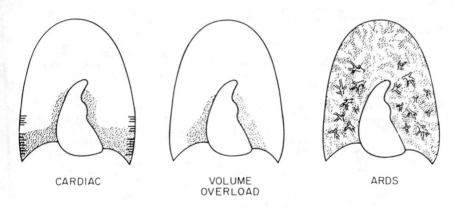

CARDIAC   VOLUME OVERLOAD   ARDS

REGIONAL PATTERNS OF LUNG EDEMA

Figure 19.2. Characteristic roentgenographic patterns of pulmonary edema. Adapted from reference 3.

The vascular pedicle is bounded by the crossing point of the superior vena cava and right main bronchus and the vertical line dropped from the takeoff point of the left subclavian artery from the aorta. Its width increases as the central vessels engorge with blood and is about 20% greater in the supine position. Blood flow redistributed to the upper lobes suggests a cardiogenic problem. The distribution of edema also varies with the underlying cause. Perihilar infiltrates with sparing of the costophrenic angles are most suggestive of volume overload (e.g., renal failure) or very early cardiogenic edema. A gravitational distribution of edema is most consistent with well-established heart failure. Patchy peripheral infiltrates that do not change rapidly or show a gravitational predilection are most suggestive of ARDS. Interestingly, septal (Kerley's) lines and peribronchial cuffing are virtually never seen in ARDS. On the other hand, air bronchograms are common in permeability edema but quite unusual with a hydrostatic etiology. Although generally valid, these rules of thumb regarding x-ray interpretation are sometimes violated, and mixed etiologies are common. Correlation with clinical and hemodynamic data is always indicated. Nonetheless, such guidelines are often helpful in formulating a diagnosis and treatment plan.

Pleural Space

Thickening at the apices of both lungs is a common normal finding, forming an apical "cap" in many elderly persons. However, unilateral pleural thickening may be the first radiographic sign of a superior sulcus tumor. Otherwise unexplained bilateral axillary pleural thickening suggests asbestos exposure. Asbestos pleural plaques occur beneath the parietal pleura and are more pronounced over the diaphragm and posterolateral ribs. Pleural and extrapleural masses almost invariably show sharp borders and are oriented convexly toward the lung.

Fluid loculated beneath the lung causes the apparent "dome" of the diaphragm to be displaced laterally and the usual "gray area" between the top of the diaphragm and the abdomen (caused by aerated lung in the posterior costophrenic recess) to opacify. On the left side, the distance between the aerated lung base and the gastric bubble (normally less than 1 cm thick) widens. On a film taken supine, a large unilateral pleural effusion will appear as a diffuse haze over the lung on that side, accompanied by a thick pleural stripe. Massive unilateral pleural effusions generate pressure and should cause the mediastinum to deviate away from the involved side. Failure of the mediastinum to move or paradoxical shifting toward the effusion is an ominous sign, suggesting coexisting blockade of a central bronchus, with atelectasis.

SUGGESTED READINGS

1. Felson B. Chest Roentgenology. Philadelphia: Saunders, 1973.

2. Fraser RG, Pare JA. Methods of roentgenologic and pathologic investigation (Chapter 2). In: Diagnosis of Diseases of the Chest. Philadelphia: WB Saunders, 1977:184-240.

3. Milne EN, et al. The radiologic distinction of cardiogenic and non-cardiogenic edema. Am. J. Roentgen. 1985;144:879-94.

Chapter 20

Chest Imaging

SPECIALIZED RADIOGRAPHIC PROCEDURES

Fluoroscopy

In addition to its utility for guiding placement of catheters in central vessels, fluoroscopy is an excellent and underutilized method for localizing intrathoracic lesions, distinguishing pulsatile from nonpulsatile structures near the hilum, determining the presence of calcium in nodules, documenting segmental air trapping, detecting diaphragmatic motion, and separating shadows of lung lesions from those associated with extrapulmonary structures (e.g., lung carcinoma vs. pleural plaque).

Conventional Tomography

Linear tomograms "cut" through the lung by moving the cassette relative to the beam, thereby blurring all tissue but that of the single thin sheet continuously in focus. Definition of the structures in that plane improves, often revealing features not obvious on plain films. In the past, tomography has been useful in demonstrating cavities, calcium in nodules, and the limits of juxtapleural lesions. Communicating vessels, bony involvement, and satellite lesions of lung masses are sometimes identified. Bullae, endobronchial lesions, bronchial compression, upper airway anatomy, and air bronchograms show up well.

Whole lung tomography can search for metastatic lesions, picking up 10-15% more of them than plain films but not as many as computed tomography. Hilar tomography has been successfully used to distinguish enlarged vessels from nodes, especially if performed in the lateral or 55° oblique projections. Evidence of mediastinal node enlargement correctly predicts pathologic involvement in 80-90% of cases. Mediastinoscopy confirms the absence of hilar involvement by tomogram 70-90% of the time. Despite its multiplicity of potential uses, its applications are dwindling, supplanted by computed tomography.

Computed Tomography

A computed tomogram (CT) is a synthesized cross-sectional image reconstructed from information gathered by passing a narrow beam of x-rays through a horizontal slice of a body region to a series of detectors. This method not only reveals exquisite anatomic detail but also provides a clue to the nature of a designated area by quantifying its radiographic density. Radiation exposure approximates that of an upper GI series or an intravenous pyelogram.

Unlike conventional radiographic techniques, thoracic CT separates structures of different radiographic density sharply from one another, even in areas where overlying shadows make conventional techniques less sensitive. Hence, CT can identify lesions close to the pleura, diaphragm, and mediastinum. It is particularly useful to investigate lesions present on PA but not lateral views and to gather evidence of extension to soft tissues or bone. Lung parenchymal disease obscured by fluid or mediastinal structures on plain film can often be demonstrated. Separation of vascular from nonvascular structures is facilitated by the peripheral injection of soluble contrast media. CT identifies mediastinal adenopathy with great sensitivity but poor specificity. Thus, in the setting of bronchogenic carcinoma, CT-identified mediastinal adenopathy should not be used to rule out resectability without independent confirmation.

Because CT uncovers nodular parenchymal disease otherwise missed by plain film and whole lung tomography, it may eventually find application to patients with positive sputum cytology but negative chest films. Presently, CT is the technique of choice when searching for additional metastatic lesions in cases of apparent solitary metastasis. Unfortunately, many nodules demonstrable only by CT prove to be granulomas, so that confusion may result unless a baseline scan is available.

By its ability to estimate tissue radiodensity, CT can provide attenuation numbers (density units) characteristic of fat, fluid, solid tissue, and calcium. CT can save a thoracotomy if a juxtapleural or mediastinal mass can be shown to be lipomatous or calcified. The ability of CT to identify lesions of high radiodensity can be put to use when searching for the calcified pleural plaques of asbestosis. CT can also prove useful when investigating solitary pulmonary nodules, since very high density numbers appear to correlate with calcium content and benign characteristics. Yet in the great majority of instances, the density value lies within a nondiagnostic range. Cysts are easily outlined, both in the lung and in the mediastinum. Empyema can sometimes be distinguished from a pleural-based lung abscess by the characteristics of the wall and the absorption spectrum, thus helping to determine the need for tube thoracostomy. Occasionally hilar lymph nodes are difficult to distinguish from pulmonary vessels, even by tomography. A contrast-enhanced CT can make this separation easily.

Ultrasonography

The applications of this technique to the thorax are limited because the aerated lung reflects rather than transmits ultrasonic energy. However, when solid tissue or fluid is contiguous with the chest wall, ultrasound (US) can be used as a probe. Thus, US can localize the diaphragm or distinguish pleural fluid from solid tissue (such as a pleural peel or consolidated lung). The cystic nature of an anterior mediastinal mass can occasionally be discerned by this technique.

Perhaps the most common use for thoracic US is to map out loculations of pleural fluid to facilitate sampling. Ultrasound can often suggest the fluid composition, since organizing fibrin, hemothorax, and empyema spaces are not usually echo-free.

Pulmonary Angiography

Indications

Although pulmonary angiography is the definitive test for pulmonary embolism, there has been a general reluctance to use it aggressively. In view of its financial cost and invasive nature, this cautious attitude seems understandable and quite appropriate. However, considering the potential morbidity of missed diagnoses based on less secure data and the low incidence of complications by experienced operators, angiography is probably underutilized.

Technique

If the clinical situation warrants, heparin need not be withheld prior to angiography, although special care must be taken to avoid local bleeding. An angiographic catheter inserted from an antecubital or femoral site is advanced carefully into the pulmonary artery using a guide wire and fluoroscopy. Central vascular pressures are measured as each new chamber is entered. If right ventricular end-diastolic pressure exceeds 20 mmHg, injection of contrast medium risks acute right heart failure.

Whether main or selective injections are done depends in part upon the findings of the preceding perfusion scan. A main injection is done if there is unilateral hypoperfusion or suspicion of saddle embolism. Otherwise, a less risky selective injection is done, guided by the scan findings. Before an angiogram can be called negative with confidence, AP and oblique views must be obtained. Additional magnification views may enhance detection of small clots. For each view, rapid sequence filming is performed as very hypertonic (1200 mosm/l) iodinated contrast material is injected over a brief (2-second) period. The volume and rate of injection should be determined by vessel size, cardiac output, and mean pulmonary artery pressure.

Bedside angiograms using the Swan-Ganz catheter should not be attempted by inexperienced personnel. The majority of such studies are both suboptimal and hazardous. Whether this technique is appropriate should be judged only by an experienced angiographer.

Complications

Injection of hypertonic contrast medium has potentially adverse consequences. For reasons that still remain unclear, contrast injection abruptly raises pulmonary vascular resistance, thereby increasing PA pressure. In patients whose pulmonary capillary bed is restricted, this reaction can precipitate acute cor pulmonale. Hence, those with extreme pulmonary hypertension are at greatest risk. The hypertonic media used also may trigger systemic hypotension due to reflex depression of systemic vascular tone. Furthermore, hypertonicity of the medium causes intravascular volume loading and can cause pulmonary congestion, especially in patients with renal failure. Suitable isotonic contrast media are now available and may eventually obviate these problems. Iodine-containing media can precipitate anaphylactoid reactions.

Mere passage of a stiff catheter can cause serious problems. Right ventricular perforation is not rare, but such events do not usually have catastrophic consequences, especially if anticoagulants have been withheld. Flexible shaped catheters minimize this potential risk. Occasionally, clots are dislodged from the vena cava or heart when the catheter is advanced. In the presence of a left bundle branch block, trauma to the subendocardial right bundle during insertion can produce transient complete heart block.

Application

An angiogram need not be performed in every case of suspected pulmonary embolism. However, unless contraindicated by extreme pulmonary hypertension or ongoing right heart failure, angiography should be done whenever surgical or thrombolytic therapy is considered and whenever the patient is at high risk for complications of anticoagulant therapy. Direct imaging of the pulmonary vasculature allows arteriovenous communications and intraluminal defects to be demonstrated. Angiography finds its most common application as the definitive procedure for investigating pulmonary embolism. To be unequivocally positive, intraluminal filling defects characteristic of clot or abrupt vessel cutoffs must be present. Paucity of perfusion or rapid vessel tapering are not sufficient.

A negative high-quality angiogram performed shortly (less than 48 hours) after a worrisome clinical event virtually rules out a life-threatening embolic process and the need for anticoagulation. Very few such patients have documented emboli in the ensuing months. Positive yield falls quickly with time after embolism, due to clot fragmentation and thrombolysis. Few situations justify an angiogram delayed longer than 5-7 days after the clinical event.

Digital Subtraction Angiography

Digital subtraction angiography (DSA) is a technique recently introduced to visualize vessels without the need for direct catheterization. DSA requires sophisticated video equipment and computer technology to highlight vascular structures imaged by conventional radiography. Following peripheral contrast injection, large central pulmonary emboli can be adequately visualized in the majority of cases. Unfortunately, respiratory and cardiac motion seriously impair image quality, and peripheral vessels cannot be confidently displayed without pulmonary catheterization. Newer equipment may help to overcome such problems. At present, DSA is a poor second choice to pulmonary angiography. However, DSA or nuclear magnetic resonance imaging may help to define central clot when direct contrast injection is contraindicated by extreme pulmonary hypertension or dye hypersensitivity.

NUCLEAR AND MAGNETIC RESONANCE IMAGING

Lung Scan - Technique

Perfusion Scan

Macroaggregates (or microspheres) of human serum albumin 15-50 microns in diameter are trapped by the pulmonary capillaries on the first pass through the lungs. Labeled with technetium-99m, the trapped particles emit radioactivity, which is detected by a "gamma" camera and displayed on a cathode ray tube, providing an image of the perfused area. If desired, a precise differential count proportional to blood flow can be recorded for the area selected.

Although the radiolabeled technetium has a half-life of 6 hours, the residence time of the aggregates within the lung is shorter, with a half-life of approximately 3 hours. Since each view of the lung requires approximately 5 minutes, six views can usually be completed within 40 minutes. The study requires a minimum of cooperation, carries negligible risk, and radiation exposure is considerably less than during fluoroscopic procedures. Resolution of defects with this combination of radioisotope and camera is approximately 1.0-1.5 centimeters for defects at the lung surface and somewhat worse for defects situated more deeply in the lung.

The injected particles are distributed proportionately to blood flow, so that the majority lodge in dependent and nonvasoconstricted areas. If an injection is made in the upright position, a disproportionate amount of blood flows to the bases; pulmonary hypertension should be suspected if an evenly distributed image is recorded after injection of a sitting patient. Although virtually any pathologic process will diminish blood flow to affected areas, bronchospasm and airway secretions can cause segmental perfusion defects. Perfusion defects occur in regions where vascular resistance has been increased either by passive compression of vessels or by active vasoconstriction due to regional alveolar hypoxia or locally released vasopressors. Hence, to minimize misinterpretation, a chest x-ray should be obtained immediately prior to the examination, and the heart and lungs should be auscultated within minutes of injection to help detect bronchospasm and rales.

Ventilation Scan

Ventilation scans can be performed by closed-circuit inhalation of radio-active gas (133-xenon, 127-xenon, 81-krypton). Images are recorded after several minutes of rebreathing the radioactive gas (equilibration phase) and while the gas is being eliminated from the lung (washout phase). An initial scan just as the gas is first inhaled (washin phase) is sometimes included to improve the sensitivity for obstructive disease. Normal subjects need only a few minutes to reach equilibration, but this process requires 10 minutes or more in patients with severe airflow obstruction. The washout image is a more sensitive detector of poorly ventilated areas than is the equilibration image and is less subject to false-positive interpretation than the washin display.

Unfortunately, only single views of the lung are obtained with a ventilation scan because multiple images require higher doses of radiation, take excessive time, and fatigue the patient. 133-Xenon is a lower energy isotope than technetium, so that the ventilation scan must be performed before the perfusion scan if they are to be done at the same sitting. This is unfortunate, because ventilation and perfusion defects are sometimes seen clearly in only one of eight views. Newer high-energy isotopes, such as 127-xenon, surmount this problem and allow a preceding perfusion scan to delineate the best view.

Inhalation of a radiolabeled aerosol (e.g., 113-indium) gives an image of aerosol deposition. Since site of deposition depends on impaction as well as ventilation, an aerosol scan is affected by many factors apart from gas distribution. In patients without airflow obstruction or excessive bronchial secretions, the aerosol will deposit preferentially in better ventilated areas. However, in patients with diffuse airway obstruction, the majority of the aerosol deposits centrally and does not provide an adequate ventilation scan. Nonetheless, an indium aerosol scan has two useful characteristics: 1) multiple views can be obtained after a single inhalation, and 2) the higher energy indium scan can directly follow a perfusion scan. This technique may sometimes be useful for detecting localized obstruction.

Lung Scan - Clinical Use

Pulmonary Embolism

Perfusion scans alone are of limited value because of nonspecificity. There is general agreement that a totally normal perfusion scan rules out a clinically significant pulmonary embolism, that multiple lobar defects together with a normal chest x-ray and a compatible clinical setting warrant treatment for pulmonary embolism, and that single perfusion defects, however large, are inconclusive. A perfusion defect much smaller than the corresponding infiltrate on chest film suggests strongly that embolism is not the cause. However, a hypoperfused area substantially larger than the corresponding radiographic defect implies the opposite. (When perfusion defects and radiographic abnormalities are matched in size, the liklihood of embolism is approximately one in three.) Apart from these instances, a perfusion scan must be supplemented by a ventilation scan or angiogram to confirm or exclude the diagnosis.

Adding a ventilation scan helps to improve specificity. Given a normal chest film, a single hypoperfused area of lobar size or greater with preserved ventilation or two or more segmental mismatches of ventilation and perfusion are highly likely to represent embolism. Many nuclear medicine consultants report high probability of pulmonary embolism if the perfusion defect is substantially larger than the ventilation defect and low probability if the perfusion defect is substantially smaller.

Preoperative Evaluation

Neoplasms involving mediastinal tissues often invade central pulmonary vessels to produce large perfusion defects. In the setting of primary lung cancer a large ipsilateral lobar perfusion defect usually signifies vascular invasion and nonresectability. Such findings strongly indicate the need for further investigation before resective surgery is attempted.

In candidates for lung resection with marginal pulmonary reserve by conventional criteria, the involved lung often exchanges considerably less gas than the noninvolved lung. Differential scintillation perfusion counting can be used to estimate the amount of functional lung on each side and thus to more accurately predict postresection disability (see p. 236).

Detection of Anatomic Shunts

Large intracardiac or intrapulmonary vascular communications will allow a considerable fraction of the particles to bypass the lung and lodge in other end organs such as kidney and brain. Macroscopic intracardiac and intrapulmonary shunts can be detected by scanning over the kidney and brain shortly after injection through a peripheral vein.

Radionuclide Venogram

In many medical centers a radionuclide venogram of the lower extremities is obtained at the time of injection for the perfusion scan by splitting the dose and injecting half into a pedal vein on each leg. Tourniquets are used to route blood flow to the deep vessels. By this method the deep veins of the thigh and the major pelvic vessels can be visualized with no more radiation exposure than incurred with the perfusion lung scan alone. However, sensitivity is probably not as great as it is with contrast studies of the same area. Occluded veins are recognized by loss of normal drainage patterns and appearance of collateral flow. Nonocclusive clots cannot be detected and require radiocontrast venography.

Gallium Scan

67-Gallium accumulation is nonspecific, occurring in inflammatory lesions of bacterial and granulomatous origin as well as in malignancy. In general, high gallium affinity is associated with cellular proliferation and high metabolic activity. Fibrotic and metabolically inactive tissues show little uptake. However, failure to take up gallium does not mean the absence of neoplasm or inflammation.

A gallium scan takes at least 48 hours to complete, resolution of individual defects is poor, and uptake is inconsistent between patients with apparently similar diseases. Furthermore, no scale for grading the intensity of uptake has been universally adopted. Nonetheless, gallium scanning may have occasional (adjunctive) clinical utility when assessing the activity of granulomatous processes such as sarcoidosis and tuberculosis and judging the response of these diseases to therapy. Gallium may also be used to distinguish inflammatory from noninflammatory processes within the lung (such as loculated empyema from uninfected fluid). Gallium scanning is a sensitive method for detecting inflammation within the lungs of patients with the acquired immune deficiency syndrome (AIDS). Even unimpressive radiographic infiltrates may show disproportionate gallium activity in this setting.

Seventy to 80% of lung cancers are gallium avid. Although some centers utilize the gallium scan to help decide the need for mediastinoscopy when the primary tumor is gallium positive, it must be recognized that intrinsically poor resolution renders a negative mediastinal scan questionable. Furthermore, falsely positive scans are frequent and should not preclude mediastinoscopy.

Radionuclide and Ultrasonographic Estimation of Heart Size and Function

Radionuclides can be employed to estimate cardiac volumes and ejection fraction by comparing differential counts at end diastole and end systole. Two methods are in general use: "first pass" and, more commonly for clinical purposes, "EKG-gated blood pool" techniques. If boundaries are chosen carefully, both give volume and ejection fraction estimates for the left ventricle that compare favorably with contrast ventriculography. The right ventricular ejection fraction is less reliable, largely because its boundaries are difficult to determine and because background counts interfere. The radionuclide ejection fraction is particularly useful to help assess the presence of congestive heart failure in patients with airflow obstruction and dyspnea.

Two-dimensional ultrasonography provides an estimate of contractility that is somewhat less reliable. However, chamber dimensions and fine structural detail of the heart and great vessels are defined with greater precision than with radionuclide methods. Estimates of pulmonary artery pressure and filling status of the right ventricle are often possible. Furthermore, its portable nature makes it better suited to patients with critical illness.

Magnetic Resonance Imaging

Magnetic resonance imaging (MRI) has generated widespread enthusiasm since its recent introduction to clinical practice. MRI provides tomographic images with unprecedented soft tissue contrast in any anatomic plane and distinguishes vessels with flowing blood from adjacent structures, without contrast injection. These benefits are achieved by a totally noninvasive technique free from radiation exposure or known biologic hazard. This form of imaging technology is based on the physical principle of nuclear magnetic resonance (NMR). Nuclei with an odd number of protons behave as magnets whose axes can be aligned by an imposed magnetic field. If radio waves of the proper "resonant" frequency are then applied, these aligned nuclei will absorb energy and orient against the external field. As the nuclei flip back into alignment, they release this absorbed electromagnetic energy, providing a radio signal that can be externally detected.

Exciting future applications of NMR technology may include noninvasive blood flow measurement and acquisition of sophisticated metabolic information that may be of value in distinguishing ischemia and pathologic change. For example, the use of ^{31}P-NMR techniques potentially allows noninvasive assessment of intracellular pH and the distribution and concentration of essential phosphate metabolites (ATP, ADP, and 2,3-DPG). For the moment, however, MRI is seeking to find its clinical place in defining anatomic relationships.

Whereas phosphorus is a logical element for probing metabolic processes, hydrogen is generally used for imaging because of its sensitivity to excitation, its universal presence in body tissues, and its abundance. Differences in the chemical composition of tissue being imaged, in the intensity of the external magnetic field, in the radio frequency applied, and in the intervals separating successive excitation pulses cause differences in the image obtained. Thus, multiple variables can be manipulated to emphasize selected aspects of the image quality. The images resulting from these variations have such labels as "free induction decay," "spin echo," and "inversion recovery."

In the chest, MRI has important advantages and limitations. Because flowing blood does not absorb or release radio energy quickly enough to generate a signal before leaving the tissue volume being imaged, MRI provides an inherently high degree of contrast between the walls and lumens of patent vascular structures. Thus, vessels with flowing blood can easily be distinguished from nodes or tumor masses, and the anatomy of the beating heart can be exquisitely defined by gating image acquisition to the ECG. In certain instances large emboli within central pulmonary vessels and detailed information regarding central vascular compression can also be obtained noninvasively using this technique. Soft-tissue resolution in the mediastinum is generally similar to that of CT. (Unfortunately, acquisition of MRI data may require a longer time than for CT, and consequently, cardiorespiratory motion causes image quality to suffer somewhat.) MRI has other serious shortcomings. Patients with magnetizable metallic implants (pacemakers, prostheses) are difficult or impossible to study. Acutely ill and uncooperative subjects unable to remain immobilized are poor candidates for the examination.

SUGGESTED READINGS

1. Mintzer RA, ed. Chest Imaging. An Integrated Approach. Baltimore: Williams & Wilkins, 1981.

2. Moser, KM. Radionuclides (Chapter 16). In: Baum GL, Wolinsky E, eds. Textbook of Pulmonary Diseases, 3rd ed. Boston: Little Brown, 1983:323-49.

3. Newhouse JH. Nuclear magnetic resonance studies of the chest. Clin. Chest Med. 1984;5:307-12.

4. Wittenberg J. Computed tomography of the body. N. Engl. J. Med. 1983;309:1160-66, 1224-29.

Chapter 21

Pulmonary Function Testing

ORDERING PFTs

Adept use of the pulmonary function laboratory can provide the key information needed to classify a cardiopulmonary disorder, to identify the origin of respiratory symptoms, or to adjust a therapeutic regimen. Function testing evaluates the mechanical properties of the thorax, the lung volumes, the distribution of ventilation, the efficiency of gas exchange, and the response of the cardiopulmonary system to stress.

To enable the technician or pulmonary consultant unfamiliar with the patient to select the appropriate tests and assist in their interpretation, it is very important to specify the following: 1) accurate age, height, and weight; 2) chief respiratory complaint; 3) other major clinical diagnoses; 4) relevant medications; 5) the question that the pulmonary function tests are to answer; 6) precautions; 7) history of cigarette use; and 8) other information that helps to interpret the current study against the background of past studies (e.g., "pneumonectomy, 1984").

DESCRIPTION OF TECHNIQUES

Mechanical Properties: Spirometry

To obtain reliable spirometric data the patient must cooperate with the technician and be able to reach maximal lung excursions without limitation by pain, cough, or breathlessness. Lung mechanics are most commonly assessed by measuring the unforced vital capacity (VC) and by recording the plot of volume exhaled against time during a forced vital capacity (FVC) maneuver. (In the parlance of the physiologist, a capacity is the sum of two or more volumes.) The vital capacity is the volume of gas expelled from deepest inhalation (TLC) to complete exhalation (RV).

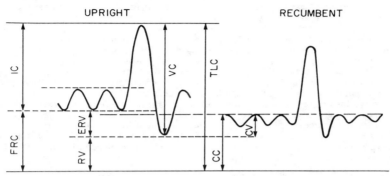

Figure 21.1. Normal unforced spirogram (left) and its subdivisions. Each capacity is the sum of two or more volumes. When the supine position is assumed (right), the major change is in FRC, which falls approximately 30% (800-1000 ml) in young normal subjects but less in the presence of most lung diseases. If closing capacity (CC) then exceeds FRC, positional hypoxemia occurs.

The unforced spirogram serves as a screening test for restrictive lung diseases and can provide clues to the origin of restrictive impairment or hypoxemia. To minimize the effects of air trapping in obstructed patients, vital capacity is usually measured by first expiring slowly to RV and then inhaling to TLC. Poorly cooperative patients may be testable by the "involuntary breath-stacking" technique.

In the forced VC maneuver, attention is directed to exhalation, during which maximal flow rates are essentially effort independent (see p. 9). When instantaneous flow rate (i.e., the slope of the volume-time trace) is plotted against exhaled volume, the display is called a flow-volume curve. When forced effort extends through both inspiratory and expiratory phases of ventilation, the tracing is a flow-volume "loop."

Flow-volume curves contain only the information already available on the volume-time spirogram but display it in a particularly useful form. The flow-volume curve allows direct reading of the FVC, peak flow rate, and the maximal flow rate possible at any lung volume by casual inspection. If timing marks are made on the flow-volume curve, the FEV_1 can also be determined instantaneously. For certain purposes (e.g., detection of central airway obstruction or peripheral airways disease), maximal flow-volume curves can be repeated after breathing an 80-20% helium-oxygen mixture. Helium markedly improves maximal rates of airflow in obstructed central airways and fails to improve airflow in diseased small airways.

Indices usually measured at <u>forced</u> spirometry include the forced vital capacity (FVC), the volume exhaled during the first second of forced exhalation (FEV_1), and the average flow rate occurring between 25% and 75% of the exhaled vital capacity (FEF_{25-75}). In most laboratories, three forced spirograms are recorded, and data from the spirograms having the highest FEV_1 and vital capacity are reported. During unforced spirometry, the slow vital capacity, inspiratory capacity, and expiratory reserve volume are recorded. The <u>responsiveness to an inhaled bronchodilator</u> is assessed by repeating slow and forced spirometry 5-10 minutes after inhaling a bronchodilating medication, such as isoproterenol or atropine. Such information is useful not only to quantify the reversible component of airflow obstruction but also to select appropriate bronchodilator therapy.

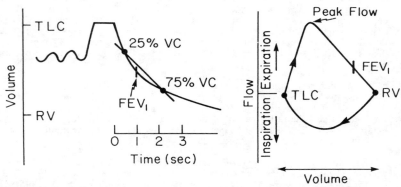

<u>Figure 21.2.</u> Volume-time and flow-volume displays of maximal airflow.

The <u>maximal voluntary ventilation (MVV)</u> measures the maximum volume of air the patient can shift per minute. The technician urges the patient to ventilate maximally for 15 seconds by telling him/her to breathe "deep and fast" at a rate of 80-100 per minute. (MVV is frequency dependent.) Because this index requires integration of all components of the ventilatory pump to achieve the optimum value, the MVV depends as much on strength, fatigability, and cooperation as on the intrinsic mechanical properties of the lung. In a strong cooperative patient the MVV should be well approximated by FEV_1 x 35. Measurement of the MVV has its greatest utility in assessing 1) the suitability of a patient for resectional surgery, 2) the presence of upper airway obstruction by comparison with the value predicted from the FEV_1, 3) degree of patient cooperation, and 4) neuromuscular weakness and endurance.

Lung Volumes: Gas Dilution and Plethysmography

FRC is usually measured, and the other lung volumes (TLC, RV) are then calculated by the addition or subtraction of the spirometrically determined inspiratory capacity and expiratory reserve volume, respectively. Two methods can be used to determine lung volume at FRC: gas dilution techniques (helium equilibration or nitrogen washout) and body plethysmography. In both gas dilution methods, the principle is similar. In the helium dilution technique, rebreathing is done on a closed circuit of known volume and initial helium concentration until equilibration occurs. In the nitrogen washout technique, the lung is washed free of its resident nitrogen by breathing 100% oxygen, and the exhaled gas is collected. The volume of collected nitrogen represents about 80% of the initial lung volume. Very little patient cooperation is necessary for these tests, which require about 10 minutes to complete.

Both methods suffer from the inability to measure the gas volume that does not communicate freely with the central airways. Although accurate for normal subjects, for patients with restriction and for those with mild airflow obstruction, gas dilution techniques seriously underestimate true lung volume in patients with severe air trapping or bullous disease, at least when extended equilibration periods are not provided. Determinations should be done after a bronchodilator trial, not before.

Total thoracic gas volume can be accurately measured in a body plethysmograph, which determines the volume of all compressible gas within the thorax and abdomen. The measurement in a constant-volume box takes advantage of the reciprocal relationship between pressure within the lung and pressure within the box, as the thorax is alternately compressed and expanded by gentle panting efforts against an airway occluded at FRC. The method is simple, reasonably accurate, and reliable. However, it requires the patient to sit within a sealed cabinet without experiencing claustrophobia and to follow instructions accurately by voice command. Recent questions have been raised regarding its validity for patients with airflow obstruction.

Impedance plethysmography (IP) is a useful technique at the bedside to monitor changes in lung volume, tidal volume, breathing pattern, and respiratory frequency. Loose coils energized by a weak alternating current are placed about the chest and abdomen. As the chest and abdominal compartments expand and contract, the impedance of the coils also vacillates in step. When the instrument is properly calibrated, the variation in electrical signals can be used to track volume changes of the individual compartments and of the total thorax. Absolute lung volume is not measured.

Distribution of Ventilation: Single-Breath Oxygen Test

The single-breath oxygen test provides two indicators of distribution of ventilation: the ΔN_2 measurement (slope of "phase 3") and closing volume. Normally, if a single breath of pure oxygen is taken from RV to TLC and then slowly exhaled, the plot of nitrogen concentration against exhaled volume has four distinct phases. Phases 1 and 2 record nitrogen concentration in gas washed from pure anatomic dead space and from anatomic dead space mixed with alveolar gas, respectively. Phase 3 records the nitrogen concentration in gas exiting from alveolar spaces and is called the alveolar plateau. Normally, the alveolar plateau rises gently, with a maximal slope (ΔN_2) of $\simeq 2\%$ per liter of exhaled gas. (This occurs because better ventilated and therefore oxygen-rich basilar units empty first.) If there is inhomogeneity in the distribution of ventilation, this slope will rise at a faster rate because poorly ventilated (nitrogen-rich) units will contribute disproportionately as exhalation proceeds.

Near the end of exhalation the curves of many normal persons exhibit a "phase 4." Its onset is signaled by a sharp rise in nitrogen concentration at the <u>closing volume</u> - that point above RV at which some dependent airways no longer contribute to gas flow. The abrupt rise occurs because gas exiting at lower volumes comes from less well-ventilated alveoli that received a disproportionately small share of the single inhaled breath of oxygen.

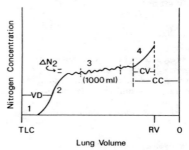

Figure 21.3. Single-breath oxygen curve. Estimates for anatomic dead space (V_D), homogeneity of gas distribution (ΔN_2), and closing volume (CV) can be obtained by analysis of the gas exhaled following a single vital capacity breath of oxygen.

Abnormal airways will cause a rise in the values of both of these tests, even when obstruction is still confined to small airways and is too mild to limit rates of maximal airflow. Hence, these tests of distribution are valuable for screening purposes. They require a patient to take a single deep breath and to exhale it slowly and evenly over a 10- to 15-second period.

Gas Exchange: Diffusing Capacity

Arterial blood gas analysis has been briefly discussed previously (see p. 32). Measurement of the capacity of the lung to transfer gas across its alveolar surface is known as the diffusing capacity or transfer factor, D_LCO. The principle of the test is to expose the alveoli to carbon monoxide (CO) and measure the rate of its disappearance from the lung. Carbon monoxide is chosen because it combines avidly with hemoglobin without producing a significant "back tension" to retard diffusion. Unlike that for oxygen, the diffusing capacity for CO does not depend on the rate of blood flow through the capillaries. At a given alveolar tension of CO, the rate of CO transfer will depend upon the hemoglobin concentration, the area of perfused alveolar-capillary membrane, and the resistance that membrane offers to CO transfer. Thus, processes that obliterate alveolar-capillary membrane (e.g., resection, pulmonary fibrosis), that recruit or derecruit capillaries (by variations in pulmonary venous pressure), or that alter hemoglobin concentration can change the D_LCO.

Two methods for measuring D_LCO are in common use: the single-breath D_LCO for patients at rest and the steady-state D_LCO for patients who cannot breath-hold (e.g., during exercise). The single-breath test is conducted by having the patient inhale a vital capacity breath of a mixture of CO and helium in air (0.3% CO and 10% He). Helium is used to determine the lung volume to which CO was exposed and to calculate the initial concentration of CO at the alveolar level. The breath is held at TLC for at least 5, and preferably 10, seconds and then exhaled and analyzed. After dead space washout, a sample of "alveolar" gas is taken to be analyzed for CO and He concentrations. The diffusing capacity in ml/min/mmHg is calculated from the initial and final alveolar concentrations of CO, the duration of breath-holding, and the single-breath lung volume.

The steady-state technique is somewhat more prone to error because fluctuations in alveolar CO concentration due to respiration make accurate estimation difficult. By collecting a mixed expired gas sample and compensating for dead space, an estimate for mean alveolar concentration of CO can be obtained. Lung volume is not measured simultaneously.

Response to Stress: Exercise Testing

Analysis of lung mechanics, gas exchange, and cardiovascular function during exercise can provide vital diagnostic information not easily acquired by other methods. Because the lungs and circulation have large functional reserves, considerable function may be lost before static tests become abnormal or symptoms are experienced at rest. In addition, some events (such as exertional oxygen desaturation and pulmonary hypertension) may only occur during stress.

Protocols for exercise testing vary widely, depending on purpose. The essential difference between an exercise test conducted in the pulmonary function laboratory and one done as an ischemic stress test is that lung mechanics, gas exchange, and relative performance of the cardiovascular and respiratory systems are investigated by measuring airflow and by analyzing arterial blood and expired gases, in addition to monitoring blood pressure and electrical activity of the heart. Pulmonary artery pressure may also be monitored. Using such information, judgments can be made concerning the cause of exercise limitation or the etiology of dyspnea (congestive heart failure, deconditioning, pulmonary hypertension, respiratory mechanical dysfunction, hypoxemia).

In many instances, arterial cannulation and collection of expired gas samples are not needed to answer the questions at hand. For example, arterial desaturation during exercise can be detected by using an ear or pulse oximeter, without blood gas analysis. Similarly, exercise-induced asthma is best detected by physical examination and spirometry done after completion of a treadmill workout or a free-range run.

Exercise testing is most commonly done using an electronically loaded bicycle ergometer or a multiple-grade, variable-speed treadmill. A formal exercise test is conducted by increasing the work rate progressively in a series of timed increments. Steps are changed at one to six minute intervals. The test is continued until stopped by an uncomfortable subject, by the development of a disturbing physiologic change (such as hypoxemia, hypotension, or arrhythmia), or by reaching 90% of the maximum heart rate predicted by age. If the purpose of the test is to assess the cause of exercise limitation, it is usually necessary to push to the symptom-limited maximum heart rate. Exercise testing is remarkably safe when precautions are taken to monitor cardiovascular function closely, especially in those patients with known heart disease or pulmonary hypertension at rest.

Other Tests

Apart from the routine tests described above, a well-equipped pulmonary function laboratory can conduct tests that are occasionally useful in difficult cases or for research purposes.

Esophageal Pressure

Mean intrapleural pressure can be estimated noninvasively with a long, thin balloon positioned in the mid esophagus. Used with measurements of lung volume, airway pressure, and flow, the esophageal pressure can be used to determine lung compliance, chest wall compliance, and airway resistance. The esophageal balloon, together with a similar balloon passed into the stomach, can be used to diagnose diaphragmatic weakness by measuring the maximum pressure difference developed across the diaphragm.

Ventilatory Drives

Ventilatory response to hypoxemia and hypercarbia can be tested during isocapneic hypoxia or hyperoxic hypercapnia, respectively, by measuring either minute ventilation, mean inspiratory flow rate (V_T/t_i = tidal volume ÷ inspiratory duration), or mouth occlusion pressure. Mouth occlusion pressure ($P_{0.1}$) is the pressure developed during the first 0.1 second of attempted inspiration after the inspiratory conduit is surreptitiously occluded during tidal breathing. This pressure appears to correlate well with the intensity of phrenic nerve discharge. In patients with impaired mechanics, $P_{0.1}$ is a better reflection of the output from the respiratory center than are the minute ventilation or V_T/t_i indices, which are heavily influenced by such disorders.

Airway Resistance

Using the body plethysmograph, an estimate of airway resistance can be made virtually simultaneously with measurement of the end-tidal resting volume, the functional residual capacity (FRC). The reciprocal of airway resistance, conductance (Gaw), is linearly dependent upon the lung volume at which it is measured. Hence, the specific airway conductance (at FRC), SGaw = Gaw/FRC, is usually reported. Although SGaw is a very sensitive indicator of airway obstruction and is obtained without forced exhalation, its inherent variability limits its clinical applications.

Airway resistance, the quotient of the pressure difference driving flow and flow rate, can also be measured with the aid of an esophageal balloon catheter to estimate pleural pressure and a pneumotachygraph to measure airflow. Although helpful for studies in the intensive care setting and for research purposes, this methodology is somewhat cumbersome for routine clinical use.

Inhalation Challenge Tests

For patients with suspected asthmatic disease, airway reactivity can be confirmed by spirometric testing before and after inhalation of an airway constrictor, such as methacholine or histamine. An exaggerated response to low concentrations confirms an asthmatic component to the illness. Inhalation of cold air and hyper- or hypotonic mists are other methods of provoking a bronchospastic response in susceptible individuals.

For patients with known airflow obstruction, causal antigens can sometimes be identified by conducting a challenge test with a suspicious compound. Spirometry is performed at frequent intervals shortly after antigen administration as well as at 4, 6, 8, and 24 hours afterward, looking for both immediate and delayed responses. A similar method (with lung volume as the indicator) can be used to investigate antigens suspected of causing allergic alveolitis.

INTERPRETATION OF DATA

Definition of Normality

In general, a measurement can be called abnormal with 90% statistical confidence if it deviates from the value predicted on the basis of sex, age, and height by more than 1.64 standard errors of the estimate. If the value observed is expressed as a percentage of the predicted value, then the 1.64 standard error lower limit corresponds very roughly to 80% for TLC and $D_L CO$; to 75% for VC, FVC, and FEV_1; and to 60% for the FEF_{25-75}. The lower limit of normal for FEV_1/FVC, expressed as a percentage, is 70%. Because the actual lower limit percentages vary widely with age, height, and sex, it is better to rely on the absolute numbers indicated by the 1.64 standard errors value.

Severity of Impairment

By convention, impairment in routine indices of pulmonary function is often classified by certain verbal descriptors. There is no universal nomenclature, and the following table reflects only the guidelines I follow.

PERCENT OF PREDICTED VALUE

	VC	FEV_1	FEV_1/FVC*	FEF_{25-75}	TLC	D_LCO
Normal	> 80	> 80	> 70	> 65	> 80	> 80
Mild	65-80	65-80	60-70	50-65	65-80	60-80
Moderate	50-64	50-64	45-59	35-49	50-64	40-59
Severe	< 50	< 50	< 45	< 35	< 50	< 40

*Absolute ratio, expressed as percentage.

It is a good idea to keep certain numbers in mind that correlate with clinical symptoms. Patients with airflow obstruction are rarely limited during normal activity if FEV_1 exceeds 2.0 liters but are almost always quite symptomatic if FEV_1 is less than 1.0 liter (provided that FEV_1/FVC is less than 50%). Unless there is a concomitant drive problem, CO_2 retention due to airflow obstruction is unusual if resting FEV_1 exceeds 1.25 liters. (Even these guidelines may not be reliable for patients at the extremes of height, age, or physical activity.)

Degree of Cooperation

To interpret spirometry, it is important to know whether the patient cooperated or whether coughing, pain, dyspnea, weakness, or other factors produced suboptimal effort. Communication with the technician may settle the question outright. However, if this cannot be done, the tracings should be examined, paying particular attention to the first and last portions. A poorly cooperative patient produces a tracing that has a rounded starting portion, an abrupt termination, or an uneven contour. If three tracings are obtained, at least two of the three should be similar. Good efforts last at least five seconds. An MVV much less than that predicted from the FEV_1 also suggests poor cooperation or weakness.

Implications of Individual Test Results

In general, individual tests must be interpreted together with the other tests and the clinical setting.

VC and FVC

Vital capacity can be reduced because of limited inspiratory capacity (IC), expiratory reserve volume (ERV), or both. Expiratory reserve volume can be reduced out of proportion to IC by obesity, neuromuscular impairment, or airflow obstruction. (Residual volume is normal or reduced in obesity but increased in the other conditions.) In parenchymal lung diseases, IC and ERV are lost more or less proportionately.

A normal VC rules out significant restrictive lung disease and obviates the need for measuring lung volumes to search for restriction.

In normal individuals, the VC and FVC are nearly identical. In patients with airflow obstruction, the FVC may be considerably smaller due to air trapping. An FVC 10% less than the slow VC is considered to be significantly diminished.

FEV_1 and FEV_1/FVC

Like other maximal flow rates, FEV_1 is dependent on lung volume and, hence, must be interpreted in relation to a measure of lung volume. Since VC and FVC are spirographic indicators of lung volume, either can be used as the "correction factor." In severe disease, RV rises and VC and FVC fall. Furthermore, FVC may considerably underestimate VC due to air trapping, causing FEV_1/FVC to exceed the FEV_1/VC ratio. Thus, whereas both ratios tend to underestimate the severity of obstruction, FEV_1/VC is the preferred index.

FEF_{25-75} and $\dot{V}_{50}$

FEF_{25-75} (the average flow rate over the middle half of FVC) and the $\dot{V}_{50}$ (the maximal flow rate at 50% FVC) are nearly identical numerically. Although clearly in the effort-independent range, FEF_{25-75} is a more variable measurement than either FEV_1 or FVC, both on repeated efforts in the same patient and in relation to predicted values. FEF_{25-75} depends upon flow in smaller airways than the FEV_1 and may be the only routine function test to show deterioration in developing airflow obstruction. Conversely, an isolated reduction in the FEF_{25-75}, no matter how extreme, cannot be used as the basis on which to diagnose severe airflow obstruction. Its value is limited by its variability and by its failure to identify those patients who will eventually progress to symptomatic airflow obstruction.

Bronchodilator Response

What constitutes a clinically significant bronchodilator reponse can only be determined by the patient. Nonetheless, on (somewhat shaky) statistical grounds a significant bronchodilator response is said to occur if the FVC or FEV_1 increases by 15% from the prebronchodilator value or if the FEF_{25-75} improves by 25%. To be valid, FEF_{25-75} values must be compared at the same lung volume. Hence, if vital capacity changes after bronchodilator, the baseline FVC is stepped off from total lung capacity, and only that segment is used for calculation. The average flow rate over the middle half of this segment is the isovolume FEF_{25-75} and is the value used for comparison purposes. A 10% response in VC signifies reduced air trapping and may be the only evidence of significantly improved function.

Interpretation of bronchodilator responsiveness is often confounded by whether the patient withheld bronchodilators long enough to dissipate their effect before the baseline measurement. FEV_1/FVC and FEV_1/VC ratios must not be used as the index of comparison, because the vital capacity may increase as much or more than the FEV_1 in moderate to severe disease, prompting the wrong conclusion. The response to inhaled bronchodilators is sufficiently variable that, whatever the outcome, a therapeutic trial with a bronchodilating aerosol is justified if the patient is symptomatic. Patients with severe disease may respond only to orally administered bronchodilators because of ineffective deposition of the inhaled drugs. In addition, corticosteroids may enhance the response to beta-sympathomimetics. Thus, while a good response to the inhaled bronchodilator warrants a therapeutic trial, a single negative bronchodilator response does not necessarily preclude therapeutic benefit.

MVV

MVV is most commonly used as an adjunctive test to gauge suitability for resective surgery. When used for this purpose, MVV should be performed after a bronchodilator trial, with the patient in optimal condition. MVV values less than 40% and less than 55% of predicted are relative contraindications to lobectomy and pneumonectomy, respectively. Lack of patient cooperation, neuromuscular weakness, and upper airway obstruction reduce MVV out of proportion to FEV_1.

Flow-Volume Loops

Information derived from flow-volume loops is particularly useful in the assessment of upper airway obstruction. With most forms of upper airway obstruction, peak flow is depressed in relation to FEV_1, maximal inspiratory flow rates are depressed in relation to maximal expiratory flow rates, and helium augmentation of expiratory flow is exaggerated (see p. 174).

Lung Volumes

Absolute lung volume at FRC is actually measured; other lung volumes are then derived by adding or subtracting subdivisions of the vital capacity. Although reduced TLC is considered the sine qua non of restriction, TLC, like VC, is effort dependent. Thus, FRC is the most reliable indicator of parenchymal restriction, because it is not influenced by effort during quiet breathing. It should be noted, however, that FRC may vary greatly from breath to breath, especially in patients with airflow obstruction and those who are uncomfortable during the procedure. Reproducibility is often enhanced by the assumption of the supine posture, but all lung volumes are reduced in this position (see p. 133).

Parenchymal restriction tends to reduce RV, FRC, and TLC more or less uniformly, while neuromuscular and chest wall problems tend to cause asymmetrical deficits in these volumes. For example, obesity causes a disproportionate reduction in FRC.

Single-breath gas dilution determinations are reasonably accurate only in normal subjects. Helium-equilibration and nitrogen-washout techniques underestimate true lung volume somewhat, and the discrepancy between gas dilution FRC and plethysmographic FRC can be used to make a rough estimate of the volume of a large poorly ventilated bulla in a patient with otherwise normal lungs.

Δ N_2 and Closing Volume

Closing volume is age dependent, varying from 10% (or less) of the upright vital capacity in young subjects to 40% of vital capacity at age 65. Closing volume is also inherently variable, even in repetitive tests of the same patient. Closing volume plus residual volume (closing capacity, CC) is more reproducible and hence preferred. Expressed as a percentage, CC should not exceed 40% of the TLC in young patients or 60% of TLC in older patients. Δ N_2 should not exceed 2%/liter of exhaled volume at any age.

Closing capacity and Δ N_2 are sensitive tests of airways disease and, when normal, indicate the absence of pathologic change within the airways. Conversely, with extensive airway pathology (e.g., chronic bronchitis) abnormalities of Δ N_2 and closing capacity are almost always present. (Emphysema causing the same degree of obstruction may have a normal Δ N_2

because airways themselves are not diseased.) The reason for unexplained hypoxemia may sometimes be demonstrated by a closing capacity that exceeds FRC. This mechanism is particularly likely to operate in the supine position, when FRC is 20-30% lower than the sitting value and closing volume is unchanged (see p. 133).

Unfortunately, Δ N_2 and closing capacity are too sensitive to be used as reliable early indicators of airflow obstruction. They do not allow a judgment to be made as to which of the many patients with abnormal tests (the majority of heavy smokers) will be the ones to develop disabling symptoms.

Diffusing Capacity

If the hemoglobin (Hb) concentration deviates from 15 gm/dl, the measured $D_L CO$ should be modified to reflect lung properties more closely:

$$\text{"Corrected" } D_L CO = \text{measured } D_L CO / (0.07 \times Hb)$$

Impaired $D_L CO$ can result from any process that reduces the alveolar-capillary surface area.

Both $D_L CO$ and the $D_L CO / V_A$ are reported to help distinguish among decreases in $D_L CO$ due mainly to perfusion defects, resection, fibrosis, emphysema, and impaired ventilation. V_A is the single-breath TLC determined during the $D_L CO$ measurement and can be regarded as the alveolar volume to which the CO distributed. If entire alveolar units are lost, alveolar volume and diffusing capacity theoretically are deleted in proportion to each other, and although $D_L CO$ is reduced, the D_L / V_A ratio remains at the level predicted for a normal patient. Thus, D_L / V_A tends to be normal or higher than predicted in diseases that obliterate both alveolar spaces and capillaries (fibrosis, resection) and in patients whose abnormal distribution of ventilation causes neither helium nor CO to reach many alveoli (e.g., chronic bronchitis).

It is important to recognize that in normals, diffusing capacity does not fall in exact proportion to lung volume, but more slowly. (This is probably due to better distribution of perfusion, despite an overall reduction in alveolar-capillary membrane at lower volumes, and to the fact that for any given volume change of the alveolus, the associated surface area reduces by a smaller fraction.) Hence, as lung volume falls, the D_L / V_A ratio tends to rise. This can confound the interpretation of a "normal" ratio for cases of restrictive lung disease. However, a D_L / V_A ratio lower than predicted reliably indicates that reduced $D_L CO$ cannot be explained solely on the basis of low lung volume.

Vascular occlusion with preserved alveolar volume (pulmonary embolism or vasculitis) tends to lower D_L/V_A, as do uncorrected anemia and emphysema. Emphysema destroys both capillaries and alveolar surface but actually increases alveolar volume.

Exercise Tests

Interpretation of the results of exercise testing may be a complex task best undertaken by an experienced pulmonary consultant. However, a few general guidelines may be helpful.

Cardiac Limitation

In normal subjects exercise is limited by the inability of cardiac output to keep up with the metabolic needs of the tissues, so that relatively inefficient anaerobic metabolism contributes heavily during the last increments of work rate before exhaustion. Stroke volume increases to its maximum at relatively low heart rates and remains constant thereafter. Further increases in oxygen delivery are provided by increases in heart rate (up to the age-related maximum). Patients who are sedentary, and especially those with heart disease, have abnormally low stroke volumes, so that maximal oxygen consumption is curtailed. A motivated patient limited by cardiac dysfunction will achieve a near-maximal heart rate. However, lactic acidosis occurs at low work rates because oxygen delivery to tissues is impaired. The anaerobic threshold is defined as the work level at which the rate of CO_2 production exceeds oxygen consumption (due to buffering of H^+ by HCO_3^- to produce additional CO_2). Hence, the anaerobic threshold of a cardiac-limited subject occurs at an abnormally low work rate.

Respiratory Limitation

PaO_2 should remain unchanged by exercise. $PaCO_2$ should remain at the resting level until anaerobic metabolism begins, at which time increasing lactic acidosis prompts a fall in $PaCO_2$. In patients limited by ventilation, $PaCO_2$ may rise with exercise or fail to decline as the anaerobic threshold is reached. Many ventilation-limited patients quit before achieving work rates high enough to induce anaerobic metabolism. As a rule, ventilation-limited patients tend to quit well before 80% of maximal predicted heart rate is achieved. The contour of the expiratory flow trace progressively resembles that of a maximal effort. The ventilation level at the end of exercise often meets the MVV predicted from the FEV_1.

Circulatory Response

Pulmonary Circulation

Normally the physiologic dead space fraction, V_D/V_T, and the alveolar to arterial oxygen tension difference, $(A-a)DO_2$, fall at the beginning of exercise. As exercise proceeds in patients with pulmonary hypertension or vascular disease, however, V_D/V_T may fail to decrease or even rise, while $(A-a)DO_2$ widens excessively.

Peripheral Vascular Disease

Even when cardiac output and PaO_2 are adequate, a peripheral circulatory disturbance may cause the anaerobic threshold to be crossed well before maximal heart rate is achieved. Blood pressure may fall.

SUGGESTED READINGS

1. Bates DV, Macklem PT, Christie RV. Respiratory Function in Disease. Philadelphia: WB Saunders, 1971.

2. Cotes JE. Lung Function. Assessment and Application in Clinical Medicine, 4th ed. London: Blackwell, 1979.

3. Clausen JL, ed. Pulmonary Function Testing. Guidelines and Controversies. Grune and Stratton, 1982.

4. Jones NL, Campbell EJ. Clinical Exercise Testing. Philadelphia: Saunders, 1982.

5. Wasserman K, Whipp BJ. Exercise testing in health and disease. Am. Rev. Respir. Dis. 1975;112:219-49.

Chapter 22

Diagnostic Right Heart Catheterization

In patients with serious disorders of the cardiopulmonary system, cannulation of the central vessels can provide diagnostic information unavailable by other means. Unlike left heart catheterization, right heart studies can be accomplished outside the hemodynamic suite and without the need for fluoroscopic guidance. Furthermore, catheters remain in place over extended periods, facilitating the sequential evaluation of therapeutic interventions.

Since its introduction to clinical practice, the balloon flotation (Swan-Ganz) catheter has assumed a central role in the hemodynamic management of critically ill patients. The filling pressures of the right and left ventricles often differ markedly in patients with cardiopulmonary disease. Unlike central venous pressure (CVP) lines, thermodilution Swan-Ganz catheters allow rapid hemodynamic assessment of both pulmonary and systemic circuits. Once in place, the cardiac filling pressures, the cardiac output, and the oxygen saturation of mixed venous blood are easily determined.

INDICATIONS FOR RIGHT HEART CATHETERIZATION

Apart from its use in critical care, indications for right heart catheterization include (1) diagnostic separation of cor pulmonale from left heart or biventricular failure; (2) detailed assessment of the effects of pharmaceuticals on preload, afterload, or inotropy in patients with chronic left ventricular failure or pulmonary hypertension; (3) diagnostic assessment of pulmonary hypertension and its response to oxygen, drugs, and exercise; (4) preoperative evaluation of borderline candidates for pulmonary resection; and (5) investigation of unexplained hypoxemia and suspected intracardiac shunting.

COMPLICATIONS OF CATHETER INSERTION

Misuse of Information

Perhaps the most frequent adverse consequences derive from the inability of the physician to interpret the numbers recorded, prompting inappropriate management.

Complications at the Insertion Site

Hematoma, wound infection, pneumothorax, and trauma to nerves and vessels are distressingly frequent when performed by unsupervised, inexperienced personnel. The subclavian route should be avoided when the patient is anticoagulated (noncompressible site) and when a mechanical ventilator is in use (risk of tension pneumothorax).

Pulmonary Infarction

The balloon-flotation catheter tip should rest in a proximal vessel and wedge with 0.7 ml of air or more. The minimum volume necessary to wedge the tip is used. In patients with cardiopulmonary disorders, compromised collateral blood supply makes lung parenchyma vulnerable to ischemia during blockade of pulmonary arterial flow. If the balloon remains inflated or if the catheter tip is so peripheral as to occlude the vessel without balloon inflation, infarction may result. In the first hours after insertion, catheters often continue to soften and take up slack, allowing the catheter tip to migrate peripherally. Constant vigilance of the PA tracing is mandatory. If a "wedge" tracing without balloon inflation persists after a saline flush, the catheter should be withdrawn until a PA waveform is recovered. As a general rule, catheters should be removed when they are dysfunctional, no longer needed, or 5 days postinsertion, whichever occurs soonest.

Pulmonary Vessel Laceration

Precipitous and life-threatening hemorrhage can result from laceration of a thin-walled pulmonary artery by overinflation or by advancing the catheter without inflating the balloon.

Arrhythmias

Premature ventricular contractions (PVCs) frequently occur as the catheter tip traverses the right ventricular cavity, especially if it is not shielded by the inflated balloon. Frequent PVCs after insertion suggest slack in the line or inadvertent pullback of the catheter tip into the right ventricle. Infrequently, transient right bundle branch block can occur during passage of the catheter, because mechanical trauma impairs the right bundle, which passes superficially along the ventricular endocardium. In the presence of left bundle branch block, complete heart block can develop. Prompt withdrawl of the catheter is usually sufficient to recover the usual conduction pattern. To avoid valve damage, the balloon must be deflated before withdrawing the catheter.

Catheter Entanglement

Knotting and entanglement with nutrition catheters, pacing catheters, or CVP lines can occur with surprising ease. These dangers are minimized by placement of the catheter under fluoroscopic guidance and by avoiding excess slack during insertion.

Valve Damage

Rarely, rough manipulation of Swan-Ganz catheters can cause direct valvular injury. Fibrous excoriations of tricuspid and pulmonary valve leaflets have been demonstrated frequently after lengthy periods with the catheter in place.

Air Embolism

If the balloon ruptures, the small amount of air injected will be trapped in the capillaries, preventing serious damage. Conversely, inadvertent injection of air through the right atrial (cold) port can be disastrous in the presence of a right to left communication, such as a patent foramen ovale.

Catheter Sepsis

As an indwelling foreign object, a Swan-Ganz catheter accumulates fibrin and may serve as a nidus for intravascular infection. Sterile precautions observed at the site of skin entry and prompt discontinuation of the catheter when no longer useful minimize the risk. Because the infection risk escalates after 72-96 hours, the catheter should ordinarily be discontinued after 3-5 days of usage. Organisms that were once rarely encountered as intravascular pathogens (Staphylococcus epidermidis, Candida albicans) are now frequent causes of catheter sepsis.

POINTS OF TECHNIQUE

Sites

Brachial, subclavian, jugular, and femoral veins are suitable. Although vein access can be achieved by cutdown, percutaneous (modified Seldinger) technique is faster and less traumatic to tissue. When the right ventricle is large or cardiac output is low, brachial and subclavian routes on the left side are preferable to those on the right because the unidirectional bend assists entry into the PA outflow tract. Conversely, internal jugular catheterization is most easily achieved from the right side and is generally the first choice. Insertion from a femoral position is frequently difficult, particularly through an enlarged right ventricle, and should usually be conducted under fluoroscopic guidance.

Achieving Placement in the Pulmonary Artery

Swan-Ganz insertion may take minutes or hours, depending largely upon the ease of traversing the right atrium to the pulmonary artery. With the balloon acting as a sail, the catheter depends upon blood flow for guidance once the central vessels are reached. Flow direction helps to place the catheter tip into a dependent region, where an uninterrupted column of blood connects it with the left atrium (see p. 14). Unfortunately, whether the catheter tip follows or deviates from the mainstream depends upon many factors, including catheter stiffness, speed of advancement, right ventricular geometry, and cardiac output. A dilated right ventricle and low cardiac output impede progress. Fluoroscopy helps immeasurably in difficult cases. If fluoroscopy is not available and insertion must be done with pressure monitoring only, the following may prove helpful:

Start with a catheter that has been flushed with heparinized saline and locked to atmosphere (to avoid clots and backbleeding).

7 Fr catheters kink less easily and give better tracings than smaller (5 Fr) catheters.

Once the catheter passes into the RV, the PA outflow tract lies less than 15 cm downstream. If more than 15 cm of line are advanced, suspect doubling back, kinking, or looping within the ventricle.

Catheters soften after only 5-10 minutes at body temperature, increasing the likelihood of kinking and the difficulty of manipulation.

Advance the catheter steadily but slowly, watching the pressure tracing. Record RA pressure and RV systolic and diastolic pressures during passage through those chambers. If the monitor has a digital display of pressure, keep it on "systole" in attempting to pass from RA to RV, on "diastole" when in the right ventricle, and on "systole" when seeking to wedge. This may assist recognition of entry to the next chamber or vessel downstream.

A right lateral position may place the pulmonary outflow tract at the highest point of the right ventricular cavity, encouraging the air-filled balloon to (literally) float upward to the outflow region. In any event, repositioning of the patient may prove helpful.

Obtain a portable AP upright or supine lateral chest film to check catheter tip position immediately after the procedure. If the site and a length of external catheter are kept sterile, a malpositioned catheter can be manipulated to a better location.

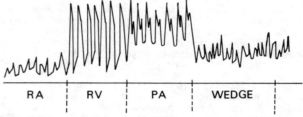

Figure 22.1. Continuous tracing from a balloon-flotation (Swan-Ganz) catheter passed from right atrium (RA) through right ventricle (RV) into pulmonary artery (PA), where balloon is inflated and wedged.

OBTAINING AND USING CATHETER DATA

THE WEDGE PRESSURE

Principle of the Wedge Measurement

When a branch of the pulmonary artery (PA) is occluded, blood flow stops between the catheter tip and the point at which the pulmonary vein leading from the unit served by that arterial branch joins vessels with flowing blood from other units. Pressure sensed by the catheter is the same as at t⊦

junction of these vessels because no pressure drop occurs across the static cylinder of blood. Since the pressure in the large pulmonary veins is almost identical to that of the left atrium under normal conditions, mean pressure distal to the occlusion (wedge, P_w) is theoretically a good reflection of mean left atrial pressure (P_{LA}). In turn, P_{LA} roughly estimates the end-diastolic pressure of the left ventricle (P_{LV}), unless significant mitral disease, hypovolemia, or altered myocardial compliance or performance disturb the relationship. Hence, the P_w usually reflects the intracavitary pressure of the left ventricle at end diastole.

With presssure surrounding the heart (P_{pl}) held constant, the higher P_{LV} rises, the greater the end-diastolic volume and stretch of myocardial fibers (preload). However, it is critical to recognize that ventricular volume depends upon the transmural pressure difference: ($P_{LV} - P_{pl}$). When pleural pressure varies it produces changes in P_{LV}, P_{LA}, and P_w that do not reflect changes in filling. Knowledge of the intracavitary pressure alone (such as provided by the P_w) does not provide direct information about preload without additional knowledge of the level of pressure outside the heart and the compliance (volume change in response to transmural pressure) of the ventricle.

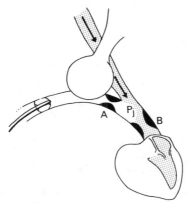

Figure 22.2. Principle of the "wedge" measurement. The pressure sensed at the catheter tip (P_w) is the same as that at the junction of the columns of static and flowing blood (P_j). A nonocclusive constriction at A does not affect P_w. However, a similar constriction at B will raise P_j (= P_w) above the true left atrial pressure.

Purpose of Measuring the Wedge

By providing an estimate of intracavitary left atrial pressure, measuring P_W allows judgments to be made concerning the adequacy of left ventricular preload, the left ventricular filling pressure necessary to sustain cardiac output, and the hydrostatic pressure in the pulmonary veins. This information can be used diagnostically to help document left ventricular disease, to establish a diagnosis of cor pulmonale, or to support or refute cardiogenic pulmonary edema as a cause for respiratory failure.

It has been well demonstrated that a central venous pressure (CVP) cannot be used to provide similar information, except in patients with perfectly normal cardiopulmonary function. Not only may the CVP be high when P_W is low (or vice versa) but responses of the CVP and P_W often lead to different conclusions when fluid challenges are given to seriously ill patients. Furthermore, "mixed" venous blood sampled upstream from the right ventricle with a CVP catheter is insufficiently blended to show good agreement with specimens taken from the pulmonary artery.

When changes in the transmural wedge pressure, CVP, and cardiac output are considered together with systemic blood pressure, the hemodynamic effects of vasoactive agents can be scientifically assessed.

Technique of Wedge Measurement

Wedge Tracing Characteristics

1) Wedge position is recognized by a tracing that develops from the PA waveform as the balloon is inflated. Although much less pulsatile than the pulmonary artery pressure, some phasic undulation should be present unless (a) the tracing is excessively damped by clot or air in the fluid-filled system, (b) the tip is pressed against the vessel wall by an asymmetrically inflated balloon, or (c) the catheter senses alveolar, not pulmonary venous, pressure.

2) The _mean_ wedge pressure must be less than the _mean_ PA pressure, or blood flows backward from the left atrium to the right ventricle! Under unusual circumstances, however, PA _diastolic_ pressure can be less than the _mean_ wedge pressure, e.g., mitral regurgitation. If measured mean pressure rises during inflation, the balloon should be deflated immediately, since it may be entrapping the catheter tip against the vessel wall. Pressure then continues to build as fluid is forced into the newly created pocket from the high-pressure bag. Such "overwedging" also risks catastrophic laceration of the pulmonary artery if the balloon is overinflated relative to the vessel size. Another cause of apparent "overwedging" in patients on PEEP is conversion of a zone 2 to zone 1 by balloon inflation (see p. 161). If overwedging occurs with a small volume of air, a chest x-ray should be obtained. A peripheral catheter tip must be pulled back to a more central position.

3) If serious doubt remains about the authenticity of a "wedge" tracing, deflate the balloon. After clearing the catheter dead space volume, very slowly withdraw a 2-ml specimen of blood from the pulmonary artery for gas analysis. Then inflate the balloon to the apparent wedge volume, again clear that dead space volume, and slowly withdraw another specimen. The "wedge" specimen should be nearly as saturated as systemic arterial blood unless the catheter tip lies in a very poorly ventilated (low $\dot{V}/\dot{Q}$) area. The "PA" specimen should have the characteristics of mixed venous blood, provided that the catheter tip is not "permanently wedged" (necessitating immediate pullback) and that the sample was not withdrawn so quickly as to contaminate the specimen with postcapillary blood. A fiberoptic catheter (see p. 169) can facilitate this process.

Hemodynamic readings can vary significantly, even in an apparently unchanging patient. Hence, it is wise to determine two wedge pressures at each time of measurement and to record the average. At each determination, the wedge pressure must be allowed to stabilize before noting the value and allowing balloon deflation. (It may take as long as 5-10 seconds for runoff to cease after occlusion.)

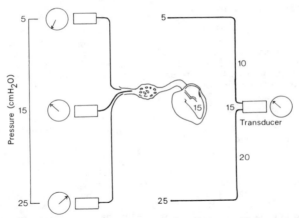

Figure 22.3. Effect of transducer height (left) and catheter tip height (right) on the wedge pressure recorded using a fluid-filled system. Because the hydrostatic column between the left atrium and transducer membrane is unbroken, transducer height, but not tip placement, makes a difference. The values shown assume 1) a continuous column of blood between the catheter tip and left atrium and 2) zero is recorded when the transducer at the left atrial level is opened to atmosphere.

Adjusting the Transducer Position

Most catheters are directed by blood flow to vessels in dependent regions of the lung (usually to the posterior or lateral subdivisions of the lower lobes). Because the catheter is fluid filled, the accuracy of the measurement of pressure depends upon the position of the transducer relative to the level at which it was zeroed. For the system to accurately track left atrial pressure, the display must be adjusted to record zero pressure when the fluid column is exposed to atmospheric pressure at the level of the left atrium. If the vertical distance between the transducer and the left atrial level is compensated for electronically by offsetting the zero, the transducer can be placed at any level, without sacrificing hydrostatic accuracy. Although transducer position at the time of zeroing is not critical, stopcock opening must be at the left atrial level. A transducer displaced below its zeroed level overestimates left atrial pressure by the amount (in cmH_2O) of vertical distance that separates the new from the old position. A transducer placed a similar vertical distance above its zeroed level will underestimate cardiac pressure by that amount. Thus, care must be taken to record wedge pressure only when the transducer remains centered to its zeroed position.

Errors may easily arise if the patient's position is varied and the transducer position is not readjusted. In any position, a point chosen in the mid-axillary line at the 4th intercostal space will suffice as a horizontal reference level for the left atrium for clinical purposes. The vertical position of the catheter tip makes little difference, provided the channel from catheter tip to left atrium is open along its full course (which is not always the case).

Dynamic Response Characteristics

An overdamped pulmonary arterial tracing (due to air bubbles, excessive tubing length, kinks and constrictions, clots, or catheter malpositioning) can closely resemble a true wedge pressure. Depending on the cause for damping, even the mean pressure value may be erroneous. A practical check of the patency of the catheter lumen and the acceptability of the dynamic response characteristics can be made using the rapid-flush device of the catheter system. After opening the flush device, it is allowed to snap closed as the pulmonary arterial pressure tracing is observed. A system with acceptable response characteristics will "overshoot" the pressure baseline but then resume display of a crisp pressure waveform. Conversely, an overdamped system will establish an unnaturally smooth waveform after a noticeable delay, without postrelease oscillation.

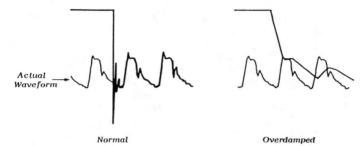

Actual Waveform →

Normal   Overdamped

<u>Figure 22.4</u>. Rapid-flush test for determining the dynamic response of a catheter-transducer system.

<u>Effect of Respiratory Variation in Intrathoracic Pressure</u>

The wedge pressure will reflect superimposed respiratory variation in intrathoracic pressure. Hence, it is essential to compare wedge pressures at the same point in the respiratory cycle. Generally, end exhalation is the best choice, since it is easy to identify and least subject to fluctuations of airway and pleural pressure.

Because many digital display modules average pressures over several seconds before updating the readout, these numbers are subject to respiratory fluctuation and cannot be relied upon to give an accurate wedge reading except under conditions of quiet breathing and passive exhalation. When there is significant respiratory variation, they are crude approximations at best. Most such units scan a 2-4 second interval for the highest and the lowest pressures sensed and report a running average of these values as the "systolic" and "diastolic" values. In a spontaneously breathing patient, "systolic" comes closest to the P_w at end exhalation, as long as expiration is unforced and the tracing is not damped. For mechanically ventilated patients, "diastolic" is best, unless the patient is forcefully attempting to inhale. With both modes of ventilation, the "mean" displayed will be of intermediate accuracy. The best display for IMV will depend on the machine support level and the vigor of patient effort.

It is hazardous to accept any digital number without confirming by direct inspection that the tracing from which that number is generated is of high fidelity. It is much preferable to read the mean P_W directly from a calibrated continuous pressure-time display. In this way misinterpretation due to damping, respiratory artifacts, mitral V waves, etc. can be avoided.

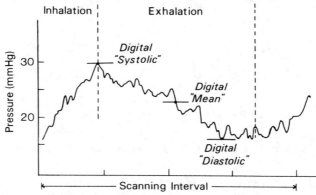

Figure 22.5. Effect of respiratory pressure variation on display of wedge pressure during one cycle of mechanical ventilation in a passive subject. Digital display scans a 2-4 second interval, selects the highest and lowest pressures, and reports an updated running average of these values as "systolic" and "diastolic," respectively (despite superimposed respiratory pressure fluctuation).

Discontinuing Mechanical Ventilation to Measure P_W

In an attempt to obviate the effect of raised pleural pressure, some authors advocate removing the patient from the ventilator before taking the wedge pressure measurement, especially if PEEP is in use. However, this seems undesirable for three reasons: 1) Abrupt removal from high levels of PEEP can cause deterioration in the patient's condition. 2) Pressure outside the heart decreases by an unmeasured amount as the patient resumes spontaneous breathing. Exhalation may become active. 3) An autotransfusion effect occurs as pleural pressure falls, so that hemodynamics off and on mechanical ventilation or PEEP may differ substantially.

Interpretation of Wedge Pressure

Wedge pressure is certainly helpful if extremely high or extremely low; however, if neither, the single wedge number becomes difficult to interpret. Different patients require different wedge pressures to achieve optimum preload. For example, a high P_w can reflect a stiff, understretched ventricle, an overstretched (failing) ventricle, or a ventricle with normal compliance and preload but elevated surrounding (pleural) pressure.

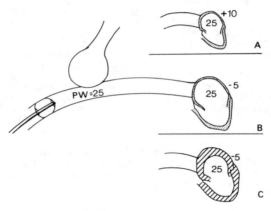

Figure 22.6. Three causes of an elevated wedge pressure: A) surrounding pleural pressure abnormally high, ventricular stretch (preload) normal; B) pleural pressure normal, preload abnormally high; C) pleural pressure normal, preload normal, but myocardial compliance abnormally low.

Furthermore, the isolated wedge reading is often of little help in determining the likelihood of pulmonary vascular congestion and edema. Although a wedge greater than 25 cmH₂O indicates the probability of hydrostatic pulmonary edema, this depends somewhat on the chronicity of the pressure elevation, the permeability of the vessels, and intravascular osmolality. The critical wedge pressure for hydrostatic edema might vary greatly on either side of that number in different patients. Independent of the usefulness of a single wedge reading for judging preload or vascular congestion, P_w is an important number to follow when manipulating intravascular volume, inotropy, or afterload.

The Fluid Challenge

A common mistake is to aim for a fixed wedge pressure, e.g., an "optimal" number, based on published data rather than to analyze the specific problem at hand. A patient with a noncompliant ventricle and low forward output may need a wedge of 20 mmHg or higher before achieving adequate filling. Perhaps the best way of assessing the need for a higher wedge pressure is to administer a "fluid challenge." In this method, 100-200 ml of D_5W are infused rapidly (over 5 minutes). Auscultation of the heart and lungs, as well as measurement of blood pressure, wedge pressure, and cardiac output, is performed before and after the challenge. A well-compensated left ventricle in need of increased preload will accept the challenge by raising cardiac output and perhaps by increasing blood pressure significantly. A modest (less than 3-4 cmH_2O) increase in wedge pressure accompanies the infusion but rapidly dissipates. A noncompliant ventricle or a ventricle in failure will show little change in cardiac output but a relatively large increase in wedge pressure that persists after the infusion is stopped, indicating that preload reserve is exhausted. Rales or a gallop may develop. The challenge should be repeated immediately if the first response occurs or if the result is equivocal.

Relationship Among Diastolic PA Pressure, P_w, P_{LA}, and P_{LV}

In persons with normal pulmonary vasculature and cardiovascular function, the PA diastolic pressure is less than 2 mmHg higher than P_w, which in turn accurately reflects P_{LA}. For practical purposes, P_{LA} and P_{LV} are interchangeable in these subjects.

Unfortunately:

1) PA diastolic pressure is unpredictably higher than P_w in patients with increased pulmonary vascular resistance, a group that includes many of those seriously ill with acute or chronic cardiopulmonary disease. Tachycardia also causes this discrepancy.

2) P_w does not always reflect mean left atrial pressure.

Even in otherwise normal subjects, P_w has been reported to deviate from mean P_{LA} at left atrial pressures greater than 13 cmH_2O. (The higher P_{LA} rises, the stronger this effect; P_w can either overestimate or underestimate P_{LA}.)

P_w overestimates P_{LA} in those unusual patients with constriction of the large pulmonary veins (beyond the point where the static column joins with flowing blood).

In some patients P_W may reflect alveolar rather than left atrial pressure (see "zoning" below).

3) P_{LA} does not always reflect P_{LV}.

Atrial contraction may boost P_{LV} and preload considerably higher than the measured P_W in patients with congestive heart failure, stiff ventricles (as after myocardial infarction), and low cardiac output states. "A" waves and "V" waves are definable on some, but by no means all, valid wedge pressure tracings. However, if present, the height of the A wave appears to correlate better with LVEDP than does the mean P_W. The A wave is also more accurate than mean P_W in mitral regurgitation, but for the opposite reason: giant V waves cause P_W to overestimate preload. Independent of its tendency to underestimate or overestimate preload, P_W still provides valid information concerning pulmonary venous hypertension and the risk of pulmonary edema. P_{LA} does not reflect P_{LV} in mitral stenosis or in mitral regurgitation. P_{LV} may be considerably higher than P_{LA} during severe aortic insufficiency, if the mitral valve is closed prematurely by the regurgitant stream. A discrepancy between P_{LA} and P_{LV} may also develop during tachycardia, arrhythmias, and atrioventricular dissociation.

Effect of Heart Rate on P_W

At the same cardiac output, stroke volume (and therefore end-diastolic volume and P_W) must change appreciably as heart rate is varied, because ejection fraction changes little with acute changes in ventricular volume. Thus, for the same ventricle, relatively high and low wedge pressures are appropriate during brady- or tachyarrhythmias, respectively.

Effect of "Zoning" on Measured P_W

For P_W to reflect P_{LA} accurately, an open channel must exist between the catheter tip and the left atrium. However, the pulmonary circulation operates at relatively low vascular pressure, and because of hydrostatic forces there is insufficient pulmonary arterial pressure to prevent the capillaries at the top of the upright lung from closing in a normal subject. Pulmonary physiologists divide the lung into zones of perfusion, according to the relationship among pulmonary arterial, alveolar, and pulmonary venous pressures (see p. 14). In zone 1 (the very top of the normal lung), alveolar pressure exceeds the pulmonary artery and vein pressures, capillaries are flattened, and no blood flows. In zone 2 (somewhat lower), pressure in the alveolus is higher than venous but less than arterial, so that flow depends upon the difference between arterial and alveolar pressures. In zone 3 (near the base), pressure in the alveolus is less than either pulmonary arterial or venous pressures, and flow depends upon the pressure difference between artery and vein.

Raising alveolar pressure disproportionately to pulmonary venous pressure, as during PEEP, increases the proportions of zones 1 and 2 relative to 3. When a Swan-Ganz catheter is inserted into either zone 1 or zone 2 and the balloon is inflated, alveolar pressure exceeds pulmonary venous pressure (by definition), compressing the alveolar capillaries. The "wedge" will then reflect alveolar pressure, not pulmonary venous pressure (P_{LA}).

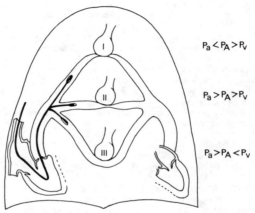

$$P_a < P_A > P_v$$

$$P_a > P_A > P_v$$

$$P_a > P_A < P_v$$

Figure 22.7. Effect of "zoning" on wedge pressure. In zones 1 and 2, alveolar pressure (P_A) exceeds pulmonary venous pressure (P_v). Hence, an alveolar artifact occurs during balloon occlusion of the pulmonary artery.

For the wedge to reflect P_{LA} and not alveolar pressure, the key condition is that pulmonary venous pressure at the level of the catheter tip exceed alveolar pressure, which it almost always does when alveolar pressure at end exhalation is zero or when the catheter lies in a dependent position. The clinical settings in which P_w might reflect alveolar and not LA pressure are

1) hypovolemia, when pulmonary venous pressure is abnormally low

2) the catheter tip lies high in the lung (usually above the left atrium) in either zone 1 or 2

3) high positive alveolar pressure remains at end exhalation (PEEP, CPAP, or "auto-PEEP")

Effect of Swan-Ganz Catheter Tip Height on P_W

If the Swan-Ganz catheter tip takes an unusual course and enters a non-dependent area of low perfusion (zone 1 or 2), the wedge pressure may rise artifactually if the patient is hypovolemic or ventilated with PEEP. A catheter placed in a nondependent region may therefore sense alveolar and not left atrial pressure at relatively low levels of PEEP.

Practically speaking, this is a minor problem except at high levels of PEEP because the majority of catheters are placed into dependent regions, and wedge pressures are usually measured with the patient supine, so that the maximum possible vertical distance between heart and catheter tip is a few centimeters. (Advancing the catheter slowly so that the tip follows blood flow also helps to place the catheter into zone 3.) Nonetheless, should a catheter tip rest above the LA in the position of measurement, it should either be repositioned or P_W measurement made in the lateral decubitus position, tip-side down.

Effect of Mechanical Ventilation on P_W

Unless end-expiratory airway pressure is increased, P_W at end exhalation in a relaxed patient should be the same during mechanical and spontaneous ventilation. However, with airflow obstruction, mechanical ventilation alone may raise end-expiratory pressure surreptitiously (see p. 191).

Effect of PEEP on P_W

Raised end-expiratory pressure, either extrinsically applied by the physician or intrinsically applied by the patient during severe airflow obstruction or vigorous breathing, has two possible effects on measured P_W apart from a tendency to reduce left ventricular preload.

Effect on P_{LA}

Increased airway pressure at end-exhalation is associated with elevation of the pressure surrounding the heart (approximated by the pleural pressure at mid-thoracic level). Under conditions of hyperinflation (airflow obstruction and high ventilatory requirement) there may be an occult "auto-PEEP" effect that is identical in its action to extrinsic PEEP but not registered by central airway pressure. Although this increased surrounding pressure tends to raise the intracavitary left atrial pressure, the net effect is influenced by the simultaneous reduction it causes in venous return to the thorax. Under passive conditions, the amount by which extracardiac pressure rises theoretically is determined by the relative compliances of the lung and chest wall. (The expression relating airway pressure to pleural pressure is given on p. 4.) During vigorous breathing, the end-expiratory wedge pressure is almost always higher than during passive conditions, due to expiratory effort, and can be misleadingly high, even when the tracing appears normal. (Suspect such an artifact when the respiratory fluctuation in P_w exceeds 10 mmHg.) Sedation or temporary muscle paralysis (during ventilator support) may be needed to establish the true value, especially when the breathing is chaotic.

The information desired concerns transmural pressure ($P_w - P_{pl}$), not intracavitary pressure (P_w). On or off PEEP, and with or without vigorous effort, transmural pressure can be calculated by measuring pleural pressure with an esophageal balloon, subtracting this value from P_w. Unfortunately, esophageal pressure reflects neither pleural pressure nor changes in pleural pressure reliably in the supine position. The upright or lateral decubitus positions are preferable when these measurements are made. If an esophageal balloon is not available, a rough estimate of transmural P_w can be made in patients who are not exhaling actively by adding 1/3 - 1/2 of the applied PEEP to normal pleural pressure at end exhalation (approximately 0-2 mmHg in the supine position) and subtracting this value from the measured P_w. This approximation can then be compared to the normal transmural left atrial pressure of 5-15 mmHg.

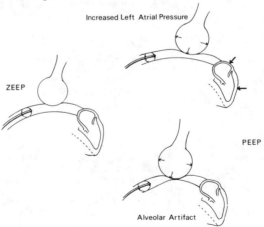

Figure 22.8. Two mechanisms by which PEEP can raise the measured wedge pressure.

"Alveolar Pressure Artifact" Effect

PEEP raises alveolar pressure more than pleural pressure and tends to decrease venous return. Both effects increase alveolar pressure in relation to pulmonary venous pressure, forcing some alveolar units to convert from zone 3 to zone 1 or 2. As discussed above, if the Swan-Ganz catheter tip happens to lie in a zone 1 or 2, the wedge will be influenced by alveolar pressure, not pulmonary venous pressure, causing an artifactually high P_w. Based on animal and human experiments, it is rare for this artifact to appear at levels of PEEP below 12-15 cmH_2O, probably because, with the catheter tip in a dependent position, its appearance at lower levels would imply a left atrial pressure so depressed as to produce unacceptable hypotension.

An artifactual wedge is often obvious because the tracing shows a very wide pressure excursion as it follows alveolar rather than pleural pressure throughout the ventilatory cycle. However, the tracing does not demonstrate normal pulsatility. If doubt remains, a lateral chest film will help decide if the catheter needs repositioning to a more dependent location. If the question persists, raise the F_iO_2, obtain cardiac output and wedge measurements, and then transiently lower PEEP by 5-10 cmH_2O until a PEEP of 10 cmH_2O or less is attained. (At this level P_w reflects LAP without artifact if the catheter tip rests low in the lung.) The P_w should have fallen by 1/2 or less of the PEEP decrement, reflecting changes in pleural pressure and venous return. If P_w falls by more than this, an alveolar artifact should be suspected. The response of cardiac output to lower PEEP and the P_w at 10 cmH_2O PEEP help determine whether hypovolemia has contributed to the PEEP artifact. A fluid challenge can help settle the question and is especially useful if the PEEP reduction trial cannot be undertaken safely.

CARDIAC OUTPUT DETERMINATION

Principle of the Measurement

The second primary function of the pulmonary artery catheter is to facilitate repeated determination of cardiac output. A sensitive, rapidly responding thermistor bonded to the distal catheter continuously senses temperature, altering resistance in response to thermal changes within pulmonary arterial blood. When the injected bolus of cold dextrose or saline enters the right atrium, it mixes with warm venous blood returning from the periphery. The churning action of the right ventricle homogenizes the two fluids, and the thermistor records the dynamic thermal curve generated when the cool mixture washes past the proximal pulmonary artery.

Technical Considerations and Potential Errors

To generate a valid estimate of output, the thermistor should sample a well-mixed cold charge of known strength. The thermistor must be positioned freely within the lumen of the central pulmonary artery because impaction against a vessel wall tends to insulate the thermistor from the cool stream, falsely elevating the displayed value. A pulmonary artery pressure waveform that appears damped or wedged may indicate malpositioning and potential problems. It is good clinical practice to inspect the temperature-time profile periodically, especially when a question of output accuracy exists. A valid curve shows a rapid early descent to a trough value, smoothly returning to baseline within 10-15 seconds of injection. Distorted curves should alert the clinician to inadequate blending of injectate with blood, to thermistor contact with the wall of the vessel, to abnormal respiratory patterns, and to arrhythmias or abrupt changes in heart rate. Information from irregular curves should be discarded.

Icing the injectate accentuates the thermal difference between marker and vehicle fluids, increasing signal strength. Although icing theoretically enhances output accuracy and reproducibility, the extreme sensitivity of the thermistor/computer systems currently available allows the use of room-temperature injectates without appreciable loss of accuracy. Although 10-mililiter injectate volumes are normally employed, 5ml volumes can be used with acceptable results when frequent measurement introduces a significant danger of volume overload. Seriously hypothermic patients, however, require the larger volume for an acceptable signal-to-background ratio. Whatever volume is chosen for injection, syringes should be filled carefully; variation in injected volume contributes significantly to measurement error. When completed within a 4-second period, the speed of cold-charge delivery has little influence on outcome. Perhaps for this reason, automated, gas-powered injectors offer no convincing advantage over manual technique.

The temperature of pulmonary arterial blood tends to vary somewhat during the respiratory cycle, particularly during mechanical ventilation with positive pressure. The cause of this variation is uncertain, but one likely possibility is that the mixture of venous blood returning from individual organs varies in synchrony with the respiratory cycle. Although it has been suggested that injection be timed to begin consistently at a single point in the ventilatory cycle, the need for this practice is controversial. Antagonists of synchronization point out that current computers are programmed to average the temperature baseline for several seconds prior to injection. Furthermore, they argue that 8-15 seconds - enough time to complete one or more respiratory cycles - must elapse before the cold charge has completely washed past the thermistor and that the timing protocol biases the output value. Perhaps the best compromise is to obtain at least three injections spaced equally along the respiratory cycle, averaging the results.

Inadvertent mismatching of the computational coefficient to the catheter is an important and surprisingly frequent error in clinical practice, particulary when catheters of varied manufacture are used with the same computer. Coefficients vary widely with the volume and temperature of the injectate as well as with the type of catheter employed.

When computational constants are correctly entered, the catheter is well positioned, and appropriate injection technique is utilized, thermodilution values for cardiac output are usually accurate. However, such nonoperator-dependent variables as intracardiac shunting, incompetence of the tricuspid valve, or thermistor malfunction due to thermal shielding by wall contact or clot may compromise validity.

Clinical Interpretation

By combining measures of cardiac output and ventricular filling pressure, important diagnostic information can often be obtained regarding the functional status of the heart and vascular reservoirs. The fluid-challenge technique is particularly helpful for this purpose. However, cardiac output must be interpreted in relation to the mass and the metabolism of the patient. (A cardiac output of 3 l/min may suffice for the needs of a cachectic patient weighing 40 kilograms.) The cardiac index (CO/surface area) attempts to adjust for variations in tissue mass. Body surface area (BSA) can be determined from a standard nomogram or approximated by this regression equation: BSA = $0.202 \times$ wt $^{.425} \times$ ht $^{.725}$, where BSA is expressed in meters squared, weight (wt) in kilograms, and height (ht) in meters. Used alone, however, even the cardiac index is of limited help in assessing perfusion adequacy. Over a broad range, any given value for cardiac index may be associated with luxuriant, barely adequate, or suboptimal tissue oxygen transport, depending on hemoglobin concentration, metabolic requirements, and the distribution of blood flow. Measures of metabolic acid production together with indices of tissue oxygen utilization provide better guides to perfusion assessment.

The cardiac output measurement can be used in conjunction with pulmonary and systemic pressure measurements to compute the parameters of vascular resistance needed to gauge ventricular afterload. Pulmonary vascular resistance (PVR) and systemic vascular resistance (SVR) are crude indices, calculated as if blood flow fulfilled the assumptions of Poiseuille's law for laminar flow:

$$PVR = (P_{\overline{PA}} - P_w)/CO \quad \text{and} \quad SVR = (P_{\overline{a}} - P_{RA})/CO$$

With pressures and outputs expressed in mmHg and liters/min, normal SVR and PVR are < 20 and < 2 (Wood) units, respectively. In the cgs system the corresponding values are < 1500 and < 120 dynes-sec-cm^{-5}, respectively.

Normally SVR and PVR are < 20 and < 3 Wood units. Although PVR and SVR are commonly computed in the clinical setting, vascular resistance calculations should preferably be made using a cardiac index. The resulting values, the systemic index (SVRI) and pulmonary index (PVRI), avoid the misleading variations of the raw parameters with body size. Significant elevations of PVRI virtually always indicate underlying lung pathology, reflecting the interplay of constrictive and occlusive forces upon a compromised pulmonary capillary bed. Unfortunately, however, the complex relationship between pulmonary vascular resistance and cardiac output often confounds the physiologic interpretation. Because pulmonary arterial pressure and cardiac output relate alinearly to one another, changes in the PVRI should be evaluated with full awareness that the PVRI is often output dependent. When assessing the effect of oxygen or a vasoactive agent on the pulmonary circuit, it should be understood that the patient may benefit if cardiac output increases, even if $P\overline{PA}$ and PVRI remain unchanged.

Cardiac output data finds one of its most useful applications in the management of disordered gas exchange. Tissues attempt to extract normal amounts of oxygen and mixed venous tension falls when oxygen delivery (CO x CaO_2) becomes insufficient for tissue needs. If the fraction of venous blood admixed through the lung remains unchanged, arterial oxygen tension may fall precipitously. Thus, depressed cardiac output values may contribute to hypoxemia, and in the presence of lung pathology variation in output may sometimes explain otherwise puzzling changes in arterial oxygen tension.

SAMPLING OF MIXED VENOUS BLOOD

Analysis of mixed venous blood can provide information of extreme value in evaluating the oxygen supply-demand axis. Blood withdrawn from the proximal pulmonary artery has been blended in the mixing chamber of the right ventricle and is therefore appropriate for analysis. Care should be taken to withdraw blood slowly, with the balloon deflated and the catheter tip positioned in a major vessel. Otherwise, contamination from the post capillary region may artificially increase the oxygen content. As oxygen delivery is reduced from the normal level without changing tissue oxygen demand, tissues initially compensate by maintaining oxygen consumption at the expense of a falling mixed venous oxygen saturation ($S\overline{v}O_2$). However, beyond a certain critical value of oxygen delivery, the oxygen extraction mechanism reaches the limits of compensation, $S\overline{v}O_2$ stabilizes, and oxygen consumption becomes delivery dependent. It should be noted that $S\overline{v}O_2$ becomes a poor monitor of changes in perfusion once this critical value is reached. Such delivery dependence has been demonstrated for acute lung injury both in experimental animal models and in the clinical setting. At this critical value of O_2 delivery, anaerobic metabolism must supplement the aerobic mechanism if energy production is to be maintained. The value of $S\bar{v}O_2$ at which this limit occurs varies, depending on whether delivery was reduced by anemia, arterial hypoxemia, or falling cardiac output.

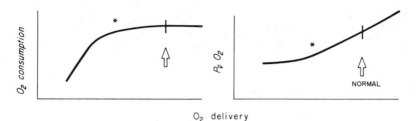

O_2 delivery

Figure 22.9. Relationship of oxygen delivery to oxygen consumption ($\dot{V}O_2$) and to the tension of mixed venous blood ($P\bar{v}O_2$). As oxygen delivery is reduced from the normal value (e.g., by reducing cardiac output) while the metabolic demand remains unchanged, increased extraction can initially maintain $\dot{V}O_2$, at the cost of a falling $P\bar{v}O_2$. At some critical level of oxygen delivery (*) the limits of extraction are reached, forcing $\dot{V}O_2$ to become delivery dependent.

Despite the physiologic importance of $P\bar{v}O_2$ as a global indicator of end-capillary tissue oxygen tension, $P\bar{v}O_2$ can vary with alterations in hemoglobin's affinity for oxygen, even when oxygen content remains stable. Therefore, direct assessment of $S\bar{v}O_2$ is preferred for clinical assessment of the oxygen-perfusion axis; estimation of $S\bar{v}O_2$ from $P\bar{v}O_2$, pH, and temperature is frought with error due to the steepness of the oxygen tension-saturation relationship. Traditionally, $S\bar{v}O_2$ has been determined on individual blood samples analyzed by laboratory instruments.

The recent application of fiberoptic reflectance oximetry to the flotation catheter has enabled continuous monitoring of $S\bar{v}O_2$ at the bedside. Although currently available instruments appear accurate and convenient, the range of clinical applications of the fiberoptic catheter has not been fully defined. Little prospectively collected data is available to define the indications for placement of this specialized instrument, but fiberoptic oximetry should frequently prove helpful. For example, oxygen saturation rises when blood is withdrawn past the wedged fiberoptic tip, facilitating the distinction between wedged and damped pulmonary arterial pressure tracings. (This feature may also help to avoid tissue infarction consequent to inadvertent distal migration of the catheter.) Continuous measurement of $S\bar{v}O_2$ should also speed the process of determining the optimal PEEP level, because alterations in net tissue oxygen flux are made quickly apparent.

Changes in $S\bar{v}O_2$ have no unique interpretation and must be viewed in light of the variables that determine oxygen transport and demand - the volume and distribution of cardiac output, hemoglobin concentration and function, arterial oxygen tension, and metabolic rate. Note that a normal or high value of $S\bar{v}O_2$ does not confirm that all tissues are receiving adequate flow or can utilize the oxygen delivered to them. The peripheral "shunting" of early sepsis and cirrhosis are good examples of distribution/extraction problems.

DETERMINANTS OF $S\bar{v}O_2$

$$\dot{V}O_2 \quad = \quad \dot{Q}(C_aO_2 - C_{\bar{v}}O_2)$$

$$\dot{V}O_2 \quad \alpha \quad \dot{Q} \, Hgb \, (SaO_2 - S\bar{v}O_2)$$

$$S\bar{v}O_2 \quad \alpha \quad SaO_2 - \dot{V}O_2 / \dot{Q} \, Hgb$$

Figure 22.10. Oxygen consumption is the product of cardiac output ($\dot{Q}$) and the oxygen content difference between arterial and mixed venous blood (CaO_2 -$C\bar{v}O_2$). Hemoglobin concentration and saturation largely determine blood oxygen content. Therefore, the saturation of mixed venous blood ($S\bar{v}O_2$) is determined by four interacting variables - a decrease in $S\bar{v}O_2$ can be caused by reductions in SaO_2, $\dot{Q}$, or Hgb or by an increase in $\dot{V}O_2$. Changes in any one of these determinants can be nullified by an offsetting change in another. For example, if metabolism changes, $\dot{V}O_2$ and $\dot{Q}$ can fall or rise in proportion to one another, leaving $S\bar{v}O_2$ unchanged.

Integration of $S\bar{v}O_2$ with clinical observations, blood gas information, and cardiac output data often establishes an early, if presumptive, diagnosis. For example, declining $S\bar{v}O_2$ and cardiac output together with unchanging arterial oxygen tension imply hemodynamic deterioration, whereas a rising cardiac output with a falling $S\bar{v}O_2$ are consistent with increased metabolic demand or acute blood loss. Initial experience with the fiberoptic catheter as an on-line monitor has underscored the rapidity with which $S\bar{v}O_2$ responds to transient changes in metabolism or altered oxygen delivery. $S\bar{v}O_2$ often falls in advance of other detectable changes and may serve to alert the clinician to intervene. For example, a decline in $S\bar{v}O_2$ may be the first indication of occult bleeding, incipient pump failure, or impending cardiac arrest. Conversely, an increasing $S\bar{v}O_2$ may signal the onset of sepsis.

A growing literature documents rapid and convincing changes in $S\bar{v}O_2$ accompanying drug therapy (vasopressors, vasodilators, sedatives), intravascular volume manipulation (diuresis, fluid infusion, transfusion), and ventilatory changes. Although fiberoptic oximetry appears to be an exciting adjunct to pulmonary artery catheterization, at present the clinical value of these instruments cannot be considered proven.

SUGGESTED READINGS

1. Kandel G, Aberman A. Mixed venous oxygen saturation. Its role in assessment of the critically ill patient. Arch. Int. Med. 1983;143:1400-02.

2. Levett JM, Replogle RL. Thermodilution cardiac output: a critical analysis and review of the literature. J. Surg. Res. 1978;27:392-404.

3. Marini JJ. Hemodynamic monitoring with the pulmonary artery catheter. Critical Care Clinics 1986;2:551-72.

4. Marini JJ. Obtaining meaningful data from the Swan-Ganz catheter. Respir. Care 1985;30:572-85.

5. O'Quin R, Marini JJ. Pulmonary artery occlusion pressure: clinical physiology, measurement, and interpretation. Am. Rev. Respir. Dis. 1983;128:319-26.

6. Robin E. The cult of the Swan-Ganz catheter: overuse and abuse of pulmonary flow catheters. Ann. Intern. Med. 1985;103:445-49.

7. Sprung CL, ed. The Pulmonary Artery Catheter. Methodology and Clinical Applications. Baltimore: University Park Press, 1983.

8. Wiedemann HP, Matthay MA, Matthay RA. Cardiovascular-pulmonary monitoring in the intensive care unit (Part I). Chest 1984;85:537-49.

Chapter 23

Airflow Obstruction

Airflow may be limited at any level of the tracheobronchial tree. Even in the absence of underlying lung pathology, discrete lesions cause symptomatic airflow obstruction if located in the central bronchi (upper airway obstruction). Mediastinal compression due to fibrosis, granuloma, or neoplasia can narrow the trachea or major bronchi to cause dyspnea. Diffuse diseases of the airways (asthma, chronic bronchitis, emphysema) usually limit flow in very small peripheral channels (< 2 mm in diameter). A clinically significant component of airflow obstruction can also occur with such diffuse problems as bronchiectasis, cystic fibrosis, sarcoidosis, left ventricular failure, eosinophilic granuloma, morbid obesity, and certain occupational lung diseases (e.g., silicosis).

UPPER AIRWAY OBSTRUCTION

Diagnosis

Causes

Acute

foreign object (e.g., food bolus)
periglottic infection (epiglottitis, pharyngeal abscess)
laryngospasm (mechanical irritation, anaphylaxis)
asthma (variant)
inflammation 2^0 to thermal or caustic injury
postextubation glottic edema
trauma
obstructive sleep apnea
neuromuscular dysfunction (pathologic or pharmacologic)

Chronic

bilateral mid-line vocal cord paralysis
granulation tissue, stricture, or chondromalacia (postintubation, tracheostomy, or trauma)
indwelling small-diameter endotracheal or tracheostomy tube
rheumatoid disease of the arytenoid cartilage
tumor of larynx, trachea, thyroid
mediastinal fibrosis

Manifestations

Patients may be symptom-free until the orifice reaches a critical dimension. Dyspnea then progresses disproportionately to further decrements in
size. The symptoms of upper airway obstruction may be impossible to
distinguish from those of lower airway disease. However, the following are
particularly suggestive:

1. Inspiratory limitation of airflow

2. Stridor

    This shrill inspiratory crowing noise is heard most commonly with
    extrathoracic obstruction.   In an adult, stridor at rest usually
    indicates a narrow aperture (less than 5 mm). Occasionally, stridor
    is mimicked by secretions pooled in the retropharynx.

3. Difficulty clearing the central airway of secretions

4. Cough of a "brassy" or "bovine" character

5. Altered voice

    Hoarseness may be the only sign of laryngeal tumor or unilateral
    vocal cord paralysis. (Although not itself a cause of obstruction,
    unilateral cord paralysis is frequently associated with processes that
    are.) Cords paralyzed bilaterally do cause obstruction, but they
    usually meet near the mid line, so that the voice may be "breathy"
    or soft but otherwise normal. Vocal cord paralysis impairs the
    ability to generate sound, so that the patient must increase airflow
    for each spoken word. Only short phrases may be spoken before the
    next breath, and the patient may sense dyspnea when conversing.

6.   Marked accentuation of dyspnea by exertion or hyperventilation

The explanation is mechanical. During vigorous inspiratory efforts, negative intratracheal pressures and turbulent inspiratory airflow tend to narrow a variable extrathoracic aperture. Exertion is stressful because obstruction worsens rather than improves during inspiration, as it does in asthma or COPD.

7.   Change in symptoms with neck movement

Diagnostic Workup

1.   Laryngoscopy (mirror, direct, or fiberoptic)

2.   CT scans or lateral tomograms of the neck and trachea

3.   Pulmonary function tests, to include flow-volume loops with and without helium-oxygen, maximal voluntary ventilation, and diffusing capacity

In general, upper airway obstruction (UAO) impairs inspiratory flow more than expiratory flow; impairs peak flow, MVV, and airway resistance disproportionately to FEV_1; and responds extraordinarily well to a low-density gas (helium-oxygen) but not to bronchodilators.

In general, asthma and COPD have just the opposite characteristics. However, asthma can have a significant upper airway component. Occasionally, stridor will be the only presenting sign of asthma. Often, these patients benefit from anxiolytics as well as bronchodilators. Unlike the diffuse obstructive diseases, which alter lung volume, distribution of airflow, and diffusing capacity, UAO alone leaves the parenchyma normal.

The flow-volume loop contour depends upon: 1) the fixed or movable (variable) nature of the obstruction and 2) the intrathoracic or extrathoracic location. A fixed lesion inside or outside the thorax blunts maximal inspiration and maximal expiration to a similar degree, giving a squared-off loop. A variable extrathoracic lesion, surrounded by atmospheric pressure, is pulled inward when subjected to negative inspiratory airway pressure but dilated by positive airway pressure. Conversely, a variable intrathoracic lesion, surrounded by a pleural pressure more negative than airway pressure, dilates on inhalation. On exhalation the lesion is pushed inward to critically narrow the airway.

PFT results suggestive for UAO include

Preserved inspiratory vital capacity with severe reduction in FEV_1

FEV_1/peak flow ratio greater than 0.6

MVV less than $30 \times FEV_1$

FIV_1/FEV_1 less than 0.9

Inspiratory $\dot{V}_{max_{50}}$ less than expiratory $\dot{V}_{max_{50}}$

Helium augmentation of $\dot{V}_{max_{50}}$ greater than 50%

The validity of these criteria depends on the position, nature, and severity of obstruction; none by itself should be considered diagnostic of UAO.

Management

Acute Obstruction

Keep patient under continual surveillance, in the intensive care unit if possible.

Keep succinylcholine, a 14-gauge needle (for cricothyroid puncture), and tracheostomy tray at the bedside for emergent use.

Administer an intravenous bronchodilator if bronchospasm is present.

If there is inflammatory obstruction, avoid stimulation but do not sedate heavily.

Postextubation glottic edema and thermal injury edema usually peak within 12-24 hours and then recede over the following 48-72 hours.

If the patient does not struggle to breathe and maintains acceptable arterial blood gases, the following supportive measures may help temporarily while attention is directed to the primary cause:

> Nurse in head-up positions
> Racemic epinephrine by aerosol
> Intravenous corticosteroids (of uncertain benefit)
> Helium-oxygen by mask

Endotracheal intubation or tracheostomy may be necessary if ventilatory failure ensues or secretions cannot be cleared. These procedures should only be attempted by experienced personnel.

Chronic Obstruction

The primary cause dictates therapy.
Tracheostomy is usually necessary.

ASTHMA

Asthma is a disease of episodic airflow obstruction that reverses partially or completely with medication. The trigger for bronchospasm may be 1) an inhaled or ingested allergen, 2) a bronchial irritant causing reflex bronchoconstriction (infection, endotracheal tube, smoke, fumes, or cold air), 3) emotion, 4) exercise, or 5) sinus drainage. Although asthma may cause obstruction that never remits completely, it apparently does not cause destructive parenchymal changes. Obstruction in asthma relates not only to bronchoconstriction but also to edema, retained airway secretions, and, perhaps in certain patients, to laryngeal constriction.

Diagnosis

History and Physical

Cough unassociated with dyspnea, either dry or productive ("allergic bronchitis"), may be the only reported symptom.

Patients often report coexisting problems with nasal or sinus congestion and drainage.

Dyspnea characteristically begins or worsens in the early morning.

Patients may report few symptoms despite impressively abnormal exam findings and PFTs.

A patient unable to converse in complete sentences has severe airflow obstruction.

Wheezing may be audible only when the patient is supine.

Wheezing together with hoarseness or symptoms of gastroesophageal reflux suggests chronic nocturnal aspiration of small volumes of gastric contents.

Substernal chest pain developing suddenly in a young asthmatic suggests associated bronchitis or mediastinal emphysema due to alveolar rupture.

Wheezing depends on degree of obstruction and speed of airflow. Hence it appears in mild obstruction, reaches loud intensity in moderate obstruction, and disappears in very severe obstruction.

Danger Signs

Deteriorating Mental Status

This is often a harbinger of impending ventilatory arrest. When patients with asthma decompensate, they often do so suddenly. A low threshold should be maintained for intubation of a disoriented, lethargic patient. Sleep deprivation, muscle fatigue, excessive catecholamine stimulation, and acute cerebral acidosis (occurring just before arrest) are likely contributing factors.

Pulsus Paradoxus Exceeding 15-20 mmHg

Normally, as cuff pressure is reduced the discrepancy (the "paradox") between the point at which the first intermittent systolic Korotkoff sounds are detected and the pressure at which all are heard is less than 8 mmHg. The paradox increases as airflow obstruction worsens. This phenomenon is believed to be due to the wide phasic swings of intrapleural pressure necessary for ventilation, which have these effects:

1. The left ventricle is effectively "afterloaded" during inspiration. Surrounded by very negative pleural pressure, the left ventricle must nonetheless raise intracavitary pressure to systemic levels. The reverse changes occur during forced exhalation. Systolic pressure falls during inspiration.

2. Although inflow to the right atrium increases during inspiration, preload to the left ventricle simultaneously is decreased because

a) A small aliquot of blood returns from the lung due to low right ventricular output during the preceding exhalation.

b) The expanded right ventricle impairs left ventricular filling to a small degree because the left and stretched right ventricles share myocardial fibers, the interventricular septum, and the pericardial space.

Hyperinflation of the Chest Radiograph

During a severe attack, "hyperinflation" occurs that abates as the severity of obstruction subsides. The increase in resting lung volume is produced by the combined effects of air trapping (the physical inability of narrowed airways to move sufficient air at lower lung volume to satisfy the minute ventilation requirement), improved parenchymal compliance, and the need to hold airways open to minimize the work of breathing.

CO_2 Retention / Acidosis / Cyanosis

When well compensated, an acute attack of asthma usually causes mild alveolar hyperventilation and mild to moderate hypoxemia (typically pH is greater than 7.40, $PaCO_2$ is less than 40 mmHg, and PaO_2 approximates 60 mmHg). Compensated asthma is unique among the obstructive diseases in causing alveolar hyperventilation.

Significant central cyanosis (implying marked arterial desaturation or cor pulmonale), elevated $PaCO_2$, and acidosis are important danger signs. However, if the patient does not appear fatigued and maintains normal mental status, these findings by themselves do not demand intubation and mechanical support; progressive deterioration in pH, $PaCO_2$, strength, or mental status do.

Diagnostic Workup

Wheezes do not necessarily imply asthma. The differential diagnosis includes

> Left ventricular failure
> Pulmonary embolism (release of bronchoconstrictive amines)
> Large airway obstruction by a discrete mass
> Bronchitis (acute or chronic)

Suggestive Historical Features

Recurrent attacks of cough or dyspnea abating spontaneously or in response to bronchodilators, with intervening asymptomatic periods

Seasonal exacerbations

Exacerbations following colds or bronchial infections

Atopic personal or family history

Concurrent rhinitis/sinusitis

Clear provocative stimuli, especially cold air and exercise

Episodic dyspnea from childhood

Absence of smoking history

Routine Laboratory Studies

Chest radiograph

Pulmonary function testing (spirometry)

Arterial blood gases

Sputum Gram stain, culture, and Wright stain for eosinophils. An unstained "wet prep" of the sputum may display Charcot-Leyden crystals or Curschmann spirals.

Absolute eosinophil count ($>$ 250/mm^3 suggests atopy or submaximal steroid effect)

Other laboratory studies as guided by history and physical examination (e.g., reflux workup, sinus films)

Pulmonary Function Tests

Bronchodilator Trial

Marked reversal of airflow obstruction after bronchodilator inhalation suggests an asthmatic component. (25% improvement in baseline FEV_1 is commonly suggested as a criterion for asthma.)

Irritant Challenge

In patients with normal or mildly abnormal function, the response of FEV_1 or peak flow to an irritant challenge (cold air or nebulized solutions of histamine, methacholine, hypertonic or hypotonic solutions) will document exaggerated airway reactivity. This test must be done by trained personnel with a physician in attendance and should not be done in overtly symptomatic patients.

Allergen Challenge

If a specific allergen is suspected because of historical features, (especially if supported by a positive skin or RAST test), pulmonary function tests can be done pre- and postinhalation or ingestion of a suspected antigen, according to established protocols. (Other than withdrawing the patient from the environmental challenge, this method is the only sure way of proving the provocative importance of an allergen.)

Exercise Challenge

Since the majority of patients with asthma undergo a degree of post-exercise bronchoconstriction, exercise may be a provocative test in patients with normal static function. Spirometry after exercise may also document the variant known as exercise-induced asthma, a common syndrome of children and young adults in which exercise is a prominent and occasionally isolated precipitant of bronchospasm.

Infective Allergens

If skin, RAST, or precipitin tests are positive for aspergillus organisms, the patient may have airways colonized with the fungus. IgE levels (usually very high), aspergillus precipitins (indicating a type III component), and a chest x-ray (showing patchy upper lobe infiltrates or shadows of mucoid impaction) may help establish the diagnosis of that disease. Control of allergic aspergillosis usually can be established with corticosteroids.

Infrequently, serious and persistent asthma unresponsive to steroids can be provoked by strongyloides, even in apparently immunocompetent patients.

Management

An attack of asthma may be brief, mild, and self-limited or continue with such protracted severity as to require maximum intensive care. As a rule of thumb, the longer the attack persists, the more slowly it responds to treatment. Asthma must be managed aggressively, with prompt escalation of the regimen if the attack does not "break" quickly.

Emergency Room Management

The most frequent mistake is to send symptomatic patients home, rather than to admit them. Patients already on corticosteroids and an intensive bronchodilator regimen would not be expected to respond to similar drugs given in the ER in other forms, but often do. Oxygen should be given, preferably by nasal cannula. Inhaled bronchodilators are a cornerstone of therapy but require supplementation in all but the least severe cases. A patient who has not responded to two subcutaneous injections of epinephrine 30 minutes apart (0.3 ml of 1:1000) or to intravenous aminophylline (0.6 mg/kg/hr after a slowly administered loading dose, if needed) is unlikely to "break" quickly and should not be kept in the ER for longer than two hours. Corticosteroids are usually required in such cases.

The next most frequent error is to not realize that an asthma attack is a manifestation of heightened irritability of the airways, which lasts for days to weeks. Patients are often discharged from the ER after a brief, intense course of treatment only to be withdrawn too abruptly from medication. The result is a patient who "bounces back" for care within hours to days after the visit.

Valuable diagnostic studies that can be done quickly include arterial blood gases, serial peak flow rate determinations, CXR, WBC and differential, and microscopic examination of the sputum, looking for eosinophils and signs of infection.

Lethargy or disorientation, obvious fatigue, and deteriorating arterial blood gases are grounds for immediate admission to the intensive care unit. A single arterial gas showing mild acidosis or $PaCO_2$ elevation should be interpreted cautiously. Most such patients will require admission, but if the patient is alert and both the ABGs and the patient show prompt and marked improvement with treatment, admission is sometimes avoidable.

A patient who does not clear symptoms completely by the time of ER discharge may benefit from a short (10-20 day) course of corticosteroids and close follow-up, especially if the episode has been of several days duration.

In-Hospital Management

During an established attack, the patient may not improve for days but recover rapidly thereafter, without a major change in therapy.

"Low-Flow" Oxygen

Oxygen should be administered by nasal prongs to all patients with less than full saturation of hemoglobin.

Inhaled Bronchodilators

Although the mainstay of bronchodilator therapy, aerosols do not reach deeply into obstructed airways and in most cases should be cautiously supplemented by systemic medications. Since a large fraction of an inhaled dose deposits ineffectively in the pharynx, the patient should be encouraged to rinse the oral cavity with water and expectorate to avoid swallowing absorbable medications. If inhaled bronchodilators are prescribed, careful attention should be directed to the duration of effective action, which varies with dosage:

isoproterenol: 60 minutes
isoetharine: 90-120 minutes
metaproterenol: 180-240 minutes
albuterol: 240-360 minutes
bitolterol 300-500 minutes
atropine: 240-360 minutes

In the first phase of treatment isoetharine or metaproterenol can,be used more frequently than this maintenance schedule indicates.

Although not officially approved for inhalation, atropine sulfate (2-4 mg in 1-2 ml of 0.45% saline, delivered by compressor-driven nebulizer) may prove useful in some cases when inhaled beta-agonists are ineffective. Efficacy must be documented in the individual, and atropine should not be administered more often than TID, for fear of drying secretions, blurring vision, or causing mental status changes.

Beclomethasone and cromolyn aerosols, intended for prophylactic use, have no place in the management of hospitalized patients and may worsen symptoms.

Steroids

Virtually every patient hospitalized for asthma should be given gluco-corticosteroids promptly and in high dosage.

Steroids reduce inflammation, help thin secretions, block a component of the allergic response, and enhance responsiveness to beta-adrenergic bronchodilators. Whether super-high doses of steroids are preferable to moderately high doses is unknown. However, on the basis of work done in patients with chronic disease, it seems reasonable that sufficient corticosteroid be given to suppress blood eosinophilia to near normal levels. The danger of uncontrolled asthma outweighs the danger of administering steroids for a brief period. One rational recommendation is to administer a bolus of 100-250 mg of methylprednisolone, followed by 60-100 mg q 6 h until the attack is broken. The dosage can then be tapered gradually to return to the prehospital dose over three weeks. Beclomethasone can be added at approximately 10-14 days, if indicated. Final tapering to the preattack dose should be done by the outpatient physician.

Theophylline

Theophylline derivatives are dangerous drugs in the acute setting. Aminophylline must be used very cautiously, if at all, with respect for its low therapeutic ratio. Failyre of the left or right ventricle, hepatic disease, and life-threatening illness all slow catabolism of its active metabolite, theophylline, whereas heavy smoking appears to accelerate it. Both efficacy and toxicity of theophylline roughly parallel its blood level; 10-20 mcg/ml is a safe therapeutic range. As with most bronchodilators, greater effect can be achieved with higher doses, but response relates only logarithmically to dose, and the incidence of toxic effects accelerates at higher serum levels.

The warning signs of theophylline toxicity (nausea, abdominal discomfort) may not be sensed or reported by seriously ill patients. Dangerous arrhythmias commonly develop at levels greater than 25 mcg/ml. It is likely that aminophylline contributes to arrhythmogenesis at much lower levels, however. Central nervous symptoms (agitation, confusion, seizures) routinely appear at levels greater than 35 mcg/ml but can be seen in a lower range. Theophylline seizures are problematic because of their resistance to standard anticonvulsants.

After loading, aminophylline should be given by continuous pump infusion via a peripheral (not central) IV line. Although aminophylline can be given over 20-30 minutes intermittently, such "bolus" therapy causes peaks and troughs. Furthermore, IV pulses of aminophylline can precipitate profound hypotension or sudden respiratory arrest.

Some published recommendations for dosage (5.6 mg/kg load and 0.9 mg/kg/hr) are excessive as starting doses in seriously ill patients, even in those without apparent congestive heart failure or liver disease. Start cautiously, using theophylline blood levels to guide revision of the dosage upward, if necessary. When adjusting for a low theophylline level, a small additional loading dose (proportionate to the increment in IV infusion rate) should be given over 30 minutes and the new drip rate begun. Without an additional load, the long half-life of aminophylline (approximately 4 hours) would cause the new steady-state level to lag unacceptably.

A full loading dose should be given if it is certain that the patient did not take a theophylline preparation at home. If uncertainty exists, up to one-half of a standard load should be given and a drip begun. One reasonable schedule is to initiate

0.8 mg/kg in healthy, heavy smokers (Smoking increases the metabolism of theophylline for several weeks following cessation.)

0.6 mg/kg in patients without cardiac or liver disease

0.4 mg/kg in patients with pneumonia, right or left congestive heart failure, or life-threatening illness

0.3 mg/kg in patients with liver disease

0.2 mg/kg for combined cardiohepatic disease

If response to these dosages appears to be suboptimal but the blood level has not yet returned, the addition of terbutaline may provide maximum bronchodilatation without risking theophylline toxicity.

Beta-2 Agonists

Terbutaline (0.25-0.5 mg subcutaneously q 4 h, or 2.5 - 5.0 mg orally q 6 h), or albuterol (2-6 mg orally q 6 h) can be an excellent adjunct to theophylline. It appears that the bronchodilator effects of these drugs, when each is used in submaximal doses, are additive, while most toxicities are not. All epinephrine-like drugs should be used cautiously in elderly patients and in those with coronary or cerebrovascular disease.

Fluids

Although the patient should be amply hydrated (2-3 liters of fluid daily) to aid thinning of secretions, excessive fluids are unnecessary and may cause volume overload. Water aerosols (mist therapy) may exacerbate obstruction due to bronchospasm or swelling of retained secretions.

Respiratory Therapy

Secretion retention is a very serious problem in asthma, in part caused by tenacious sputum. Unfortunately, chest percussion and postural drainage are relatively ineffective and poorly tolerated until a measure of bronchospasm has been relieved (usually the second or third day). Until then, coaching to cough, inhaled bronchodilators, and oxygen therapy are the limits of useful RT services. IPPB is relatively contraindicated in asthmatic patients, due to induction of air trapping.

Other Medications

Infective causes for bronchospasm must be treated. Fever and a profusion of polys and organisms on sputum Gram stain are the best indicators. Blood leukocyte count may be elevated due to stress, catecholamines, or steroids. While patchy micronodular infiltrates that result from plugged bronchi or interstitial edema are common in uncomplicated attacks of asthma, localized consolidation suggests pneumonia or bronchopulmonary aspergillosis.

Beta-blockers, especially such nonselective drugs as propranolol, may precipitate bronchospasm in labile asthmatics. Adverse effects usually occur soon after starting therapy and often at low dosage. Some increase in bronchospasm is likely in most patients, which may or may not be compensated for by coadministration of a beta$_2$-stimulator.

Hence, beta-blockers must be avoided if at all possible. If a trial of beta-blockers is justified because of intractable hypertension or angina, a relatively selective beta$_1$-blocker (e.g., metoprolol) may be preferable to propranolol. The first doses should be small and administered under close observation.

Calcium channel blockers. Anecdotal reports suggest that calcium channel blockers (e.g., nifedepine) may be helpful in certain patients. At the present time this area of investigation is still too unsettled to warrant any recommendation for their use.

The administration of hypnotics or sedatives may precipitate ventilatory arrest in these fatigued patients and are contraindicated.

Mechanical Ventilation

Unlike many COPD patients, asthmatics tend to sustain adequate alveolar ventilation during attacks until sudden decompensation occurs. Furthermore, they tolerate mechanical ventilation with less risk of complications and generally can be weaned as fast as their acute bronchospasm reverses. Respiratory muscles may consume large quantities of oxygen during an attack, and fatigue is a constant risk. Mechanical support may afford the rest needed for recovery and compensation. For these reasons, the threshold to intervene with intubation and mechanical ventilation should be set somewhat lower than when managing COPD. Mental status or blood gas deterioration that occurs despite aggressive medical therapy is an important indication for ventilator support.

CHRONIC OBSTRUCTIVE PULMONARY DISEASE (COPD)

The obstructive diseases associated with cigarette smoking (emphysema and chronic bronchitis) cause similar disability and often coexist. Nonetheless, they are quite different processes. Emphysema destroys the alveolar surface membrane and vessels, reducing elastic recoil but leaving the airways morphologically intact; emphysematous obstruction of the airway is a functional, not an anatomic, problem. Conversely, chronic bronchitis causes airway damage, bronchospasm, and sputum production but leaves the parenchyma unaffected. In both, accelerated loss of ventilatory reserve abates as smoking is stopped.

Diagnosis

Emphysema vs. Chronic Bronchitis

Pure emphysema is distinguishable from chronic bronchitis by the following:

CXR: Bullae, hyperlucency, diminished peripheral vascular markings, and increased lung volume are seen in emphysema. These findings differ from the increased bronchovascular markings and more normal lung volumes of chronic bronchitis.

History: Patients with pure emphysema produce little or no sputum. Conversely, chronic bronchitis is defined as an airway disease in which there is habitual morning sputum production (although that characteristic is shared by other airway diseases, such as sinusitis and bronchiectasis).

Emphysemic patients tend to be breathless with minimal exertion but usually do not enter the hospital with exacerbations of their disease until the terminal phase. In contrast, chronic bronchitics are often relatively indifferent to their obstruction but decompensate more frequently.

The caricatures of emphysemics as "pink puffers" and chronic bronchitics as "blue bloaters" are overdrawn. Emphysema tends to destroy capillaries and alveolar septae in proportion to one another, preserving near normal gas exchange, whereas bronchitis produces extensive $\dot{V}/\dot{Q}$ mismatch and hypoxemia. However, many patients with advanced emphysema do not have vigorous ventilatory drives, whereas some with chronic bronchitis do.   Thus, some emphysemics with moderate obstruction retain CO_2 and are not breathless, whereas occasional patients with chronic bronchitis are "blue puffers."

Pulmonary function tests: When corrected for lung volume, impaired diffusing capacity (D_L/V_A) and increased parenchymal compliance are highly characteristic of emphysema but not of chronic bronchitis.

Physical findings: Emphysemic patients tend to be more malnourished than patients with chronic bronchitis. Pulmonary hypertension marks the end stage of both diseases, but for different reasons.   In pure emphysema, pulmonary capillaries are destroyed, but normal saturation of arterial blood is preserved.   In chronic bronchitis, pulmonary hypertension develops earlier, due to persistent alveolar hypoxia. Hence, cor pulmonale in a patient with bronchitis and hypoxemia may be partially reversible with supplemental oxygen.   Cor pulmonale in emphysema is an ominous sign, responding poorly to therapy unless hypoxemia coexists. Even when relatively symptom-free, both kinds of patient tend to have tachycardia at rest.

Associated Problems

Hyperinflation: Hyperinflation helps airflow but increases the elastic work of breathing.   More importantly, the inspiratory musculature is placed at a serious mechanical disadvantage.

Bullae are usually distributed in the upper lobes. Lower lobe bullae suggest alpha$_1$-antitrypsin deficiency. Bullae may fill when the surrounding parenchyma is infiltrated, simulating cavities or lung abscesses. However, distinction by chest film can usually be made easily, and the prognosis is much better than for abscess.

Abnormal airways and bullae occasionally colonize with aspergillus, atypical mycobacteria, or nocardia.

Infection and CHF are often difficult to distinguish from one another or from chronic scarring because the parenchyma is hyperinflated and disordered and because the heart may appear small despite enlargement.

Diagnostic Workup

History, CXR, ECG
Pulmonary function tests
Arterial blood gases

Sputum and blood for eosinophils
Sputum for Gram stain and culture
Alpha$_1$-antitrypsin level, pilocarpine iontophoresis (cystic fibrosis), and
  bronchography in young patients (less than 40 yrs) with otherwise
  unexplained disease

Management

The exact cause for many exacerbations of COPD remains unknown. Numerous patients with severe disease blame climatic changes. However, treatable causes for deterioration must be sought, which include

Medication withdrawal
Infection of sinuses or bronchi
Pneumonia
Allergy (check sputum for eosinophils and polys)
Congestive heart failure or arrhythmia
Pneumothorax
Electrolyte disturbance
Cough fractures of ribs (check oblique CXR or bone scan)
Abdominal complaints (constipation, theophylline, air swallowing, peptic disease)
Musculoskeletal problems (including thoracic and abdominal muscle strain due to coughing or forceful breathing)

Oxygen Therapy

While true that high inspired fractions of oxygen may cause catastrophic blunting of drive in susceptible individuals, administration of the correct low fraction can be life saving. In hypoxic patients, oxygen improves alertness and muscular function and helps relieve cor pulmonale. (For this latter reason oxygen is a good diuretic in such cases.)

Although Venturi masks deliver a fixed F_iO_2, nasal prongs are more comfortable for patients with dyspnea and allow expectoration without interrupting the flow of oxygen.

Any patient relieved of hypoxemia will retain slightly more CO_2 because hypercapneic drive and hypoxic drive are both reduced as supplemental oxygen is given. Two general rules are useful:

1. Patients at risk to retain excessive CO_2 are those who already manifest elevated $PaCO_2$ before O_2 therapy is initiated.

2.   With "low-flow" oxygen, the rise in $PaCO_2$ is generally less than 10 mmHg and usually occurs within the first hour of oxygen administration.

Thus, rather than withhold oxygen, the appropriate strategy is to raise PaO_2 to 55-60 mmHg, to watch the patient closely for signs of obtundation, to obtain blood gases at 20-30 minutes, and to adjust the oxygen flow rate accordingly. The proper endpoint is an acceptable PaO_2, documented by blood gas analysis.

Medication Regimen

Bronchodilator therapy is similar to that described for asthma (see p. 181). However, it is necessary to remember that the reversible component in COPD is usually small, and the patients are more fragile. Reestablishing proper nutrition, fluid/electrolyte balance, oxygen therapy, and respiratory therapy assumes greater importance.

Whether to give antibiotics or corticosteroids is partly determined by the sputum smear. Sputum with polys and stainable organisms should be treated with an appropriate antibiotic, while sputum eosinophilia suggests the utility of corticosteroids. If no organism is seen, a virus or mycoplasma is a possible cause of the exacerbation. Legionella is recognized as a community-acquired pathogen with increasing frequency.

A patient who continues to do poorly despite initial measures should probably receive a trial of corticosteroids for at least 4 days. A reasonable schedule is 0.5 mg/kg q 6 h during the crises, with rapid tapering thereafter. Given steroids, some patients improve both baseline function and response to bronchodilators. Such persons have been termed "hidden asthmatics."

Management of fluids and diuretics is difficult, especially in the presence of cor pulmonale. Without florid intravascular volume depletion or overload, administration of fluids or diuretics should be gentle.

Use of Beta-Blockers in COPD

Angina, hypertension, and COPD frequently coexist. The bronchospastic component of COPD may worsen as beta-blockers are added to the regimen, especially in patients with sputum or blood eosinophilia and in those with good responses to inhaled bronchodilators or corticosteroids. Metoprolol, a semiselective $beta_1$-blocker, appears to cause less spasm than propranolol. When combined with a $beta_2$-stimulator, such as terbutaline, the majority of patients with COPD can tolerate metoprolol without significant loss of lung function. Nonetheless, therapy must begin cautiously, with documentation of effect by lung function testing. Indiscriminate use of beta-blockers (especially propranolol) is hazardous.

Respiratory Therapy

Respiratory therapy (RT) assumes a critical role in the management of hospitalized patients. Most problems can be reversed with relief of hypoxemia, treatment of infection or fluid overload, and improved secretion clearance with the RT techniques of coughing, deep breathing, and intensified bronchodilator therapy. The patient must be actively stimulated to cough, using endotracheal suctioning if necessary. Chest percussion and postural drainage are quite effective when tolerated. However, no physiotherapy technique should be continued unless its efficacy can be documented.

Intubation and Mechanical Ventilation

Intubation and mechanical ventilation must be avoided whenever possible for the following reasons:

1. Most patients without advanced cor pulmonale tolerate moderate hypoxemia and mild acidosis well.

2. An effective cough does a much better job of clearing the peripheral airways than endotracheal intubation and suctioning.

3. COPD patients are at particular risk for the complications of mechanical ventilation and are exceptionally difficult to wean, due to high work-cost of breathing, weakness, and muscular discoordination.

Indications for intubation include

1. deteriorating mental status

2. loss of effective cough (with retained secretions in central airways)

3. progressive respiratory acidosis despite aggressive medical and respiratory therapy

If mechanical assistance is necessary:

1. Care should be taken not to overventilate with respect to the previous chronic state of CO_2 retention, a condition signalled by the sudden development of apparent metabolic alkalosis when mechanical assistance is begun.

2. Test for the "auto-PEEP" effect. Most acutely ill patients with severe airflow obstruction will require high lung volumes to accomplish the ventilation they require. The consequence is positive alveolar pressure at end expiration. This auto-PEEP effect is not only associated with cardiovascular consequences but also with increased work of breathing. Air trapping-related increases in end-expiratory alveolar pressure almost certainly occur during spontaneous breathing as well.

3. IMV and pressure support may be particularly useful methods of weaning because they allow gradual resumption of the breathing workload.

Arrhythmias

Atrial and ventricular arrhythmias of all types are common, due to right atrial stretch, catecholamine release, and hypoxemia. Multifocal atrial tachycardia (chaotic but coordinated atrial contraction originating from at least three pacemaking foci) is a characteristic rhythm that often responds to nothing except relief of metabolic derangement and respiratory failure. In certain cases a calcium channel blocker, such as verapamil, can be effective in slowing the rate.

Nutrition

The ability of the patient with COPD to cope with the respiratory work load depends on the strength and endurance of the ventilatory pump. Maintaining adequate nutrition is vital. Diaphragmatic bulk parallels body weight. Although it is possible to raise CO_2 production by overfeeding carbohydrate calories, this seldom presents a problem in hospitalized patients who are able to eat normally. Rather, attention should focus on providing adequate nutrition to these patients ($\approx$ 2000 calories daily).

SUGGESTED READINGS

1. Clark TJ, Godfrey S. Asthma, 2nd ed. London: Chapman and Hall, 1983.

2. Hiller FC, Wilson FJ Jr. Evaluation and management of acute asthma. Med. Clin. North Am. 1983;67:669-84.

3. Hodgkin JE, et al. Chronic Obstructive Airway Diseases. Park Ridge Illinois: American College of Chest Physicians, 1979.

4. Kryger M, et al. Diagnosis of obstruction of the upper and central airways. Am. J. Med. 1976;61:85-93.

5. Lertzman MM, Cherniack RM. Rehabilitation of patients with chronic obstructive pulmonary disease. Am. Rev. Respir. Dis. 1976;114:1145-65.

6. Niewoehner DE. Clinical aspects of chronic airflow obstruction (Chapter 45). In: Baun GL, Wolinsky E, eds. Textbook of Pulmonary Diseases, 3rd ed. Boston: Little Brown, 1983:915-48.

7. Pepe PE, Marini JJ. Occult positive end-expiratory pressure in mechanically ventilated patients with airflow obstruction. The auto-PEEP effect. Am. Rev. Respir. Dis. 1982;126:166-70.

8. Petty TL. Improving patients with advanced chronic airflow obstruction. Chest 1983;83:713-14.

9. Proctor DF. The upper airways. The larynx and trachea. Am. Rev. Respir. Dis. 1977;115:315-42.

Chapter 24

Aspiration

Aspirated foreign materials may occlude the air passage or induce pneumonitis. For descriptive purposes, aspirated substances can be classified as ingested liquids and solids, oropharyngeal secretions, or gastric contents.

DIAGNOSIS

Foreign Liquids and Solids

Large solid objects usually arrest at the supraglottic level. Differentiation of aspirated from swallowed flat objects (such as coins) can often be made radiographically; orientation is in the sagittal plane for objects in the trachea and in the coronal plane for those in the esophagus.

Small discrete objects, such as peanuts, can nearly occlude a major bronchus. Inspiratory-expiratory films help uncover obstructive hyperinflation.

Irritants of any kind can cause bronchospasm and wheezing.

Food aspiration is particularly common when simultaneously laughing and attempting to chew. Hence, the restaurant is a common setting for the "cafe coronary."

Adult hydrocarbon aspiration has been seen frequently in recent years due to the practice of syphoning gasoline. Hydrocarbon aspiration causes intense inflammation, frequently with pneumatocele formation and superinfection.

Aspirated particulates, especially organic vegetable matter and lipids, produce an intense chemical pneumonitis. Mineral oil and oily nose drops (which are sniffed) are broken down into injurious fatty acids by lung lipases and can produce bronchial inflammation and chronic pneumonitis (often asymptomatic). The oil of an aspirated peanut is notorious for producing a severe local reaction.

With acutely advancing obtundation, the protective reflexes guarding the lung are lost in a cephalocaudal progression. Thus, gag, laryngeal, and cough reflexes are lost in that order and return in the reverse sequence. On this basis an adequate gag reflex would seem to be good justification for restarting oral feedings. Unfortunately, this is not a reliable rule; the presence or absence of a gag reflex has little predictive value for the risk of aspiration in other settings (such as neuromuscular disease).

Barium aspiration is relatively innocuous. Conversely, a large volume of aspirated hypertonic contrast media (such as Gastrografin) may cause pulmonary edema or bronchospasm.

Oropharyngeal Secretions

Although aspiration during waking hours occurs infrequently, inhalation of small amounts of oropharyngeal or nasopharyngeal secretions during sleep is almost universal. Bacterial pneumonitis usually develops by such a mechanism.

Although sometimes regarded as protection against this form of contamination, an endotracheal tube can actually serve as a conduit to the lung. Small quantities of oropharyngeal secretions migrate externally along channels formed by the folds of the tube cuff.

Gastric Contents

Esophageal reflux is common in hospitalized patients, especially in the fully recumbent position. Nasogastric tubes may render both swallowing and the esophagogastric sphincter dysfunctional, markedly increasing the risk of aspiration, especially if bolus feedings are given. During depressed states of consciousness (sleep, coma, anesthesia), gastric contents may enter the tracheobronchial tree without provoking cough. (Dye instilled into the stomachs of preoperative patients enters the trachea in about 15-20% of cases.) Aspiration can take the form of overt vomiting or unobtrusive regurgitation that escapes clinical notice.

The reaction incited by gastric contents or tube feedings depends upon osmolality, pH, lipid content, etc. and may vary from a clinically inapparent response to intense bronchospasm and ARDS. Mendelson's syndrome is the eponym for massive aspiration of acidic gastric contents, with the development of noncardiogenic edema. A pH below 2.5 is an important and perhaps critical factor. Digestive products and gastric enzymes buffer pH but cause other chemical injury.

Massive unilateral or exclusively basilar infiltration should raise suspicion of gastric aspiration.

Repeated aspiration of small amounts of gastric contents may be an occult phenomenon, presenting as chronic cough, hoarseness, asthma, or basilar fibrosis.

Recurrent pneumonia in a basilar location, especially the right lower lobe, is often due to aspiration.

DIAGNOSTIC WORKUP

If a definite history of solid foreign body aspiration is obtained and the patient is not in immediate respiratory distress, inspiratory and expiratory chest films, arterial blood gases, laryngoscopy, and bronchoscopy should be performed. Lateral neck views, as well as computerized and/or conventional tomography of the upper airway and major bronchi, may be helpful prior to endoscopic procedures. Large particulate aspiration (e.g., food) deserves fiberoptic bronchoscopy to look for bronchial occlusion.

The swallowing mechanism can be evaluated noninvasively by lateral neck tomograms, barium swallow (looking for hang-up of barium in the valleculae, Zenker's diverticulum, abnormal esophageal strictures, or dilatations), and, most elegantly, by a cineswallow. Panendoscopy of the larynx and esophagus may be useful.

The suspicion of esophageal reflux should be investigated by the usual radiographic and GI techniques.

MANAGEMENT

Solid Foreign Objects

Solid foreign objects should be removed expeditiously since delay invites postobstructive pneumonia and stricture. The fiberoptic bronchoscope has a variety of specialized forceps to aid extraction. If fiberoptic bronchoscopy is unable to remove the object, rigid bronchoscopy is indicated. Occasionally, removal by open bronchotomy or segmental resection is necessary.

Food and Gastric Contents

Prophylaxis

Aspiration of food and gastric contents is one of the most dangerous and preventable complications of serious illness.

Caution is essential; the gag reflex of all seriously ill patients who will ingest foods or liquids should first be tested. Those with a poor gag and any patient with a neck mass, tracheostomy, or recent CVA should be given plain water to drink under observation before ordering the diet.

In general, motor disorders of swallowing are screened well by liquids. (Coughing indicates aspiration.) Semi-solids are easier to swallow than are liquids, but carry a higher risk of complications if aspiration does occur. Therefore, patients recovering from surgery, those with new tracheostomies, and those freshly extubated of endotracheal or nasogastric tubes should progress from "clear liquids," to "full liquids," to "solids" over several days, as they demonstrate the abililty to handle them.

Enteral alimentation can be accomplished by bolus delivery into the stomach or by continuous "drip" infusion of nutrients into the stomach or duodenum. Aspiration is always a risk with either method, but the greater hazard is with the intermittent technique. Patients who are to begin tube feedings should have peristaltic sounds. Before starting, it is good practice to pass a standard NG tube into the stomach to decompress it and to check for fluid retention. A residual greater than 100 ml suggests the possibility of gastric hypomotility or outlet obstruction. The residual must be rechecked 1 hour after the residual is returned to the stomach. Whenever bolus tube feedings are intended, a 200 ml water load should be given, checking residuals at 1/2 and 1 hour.

If the patient passes these tests, the large NG tube is withdrawn and replaced with a small, pliable feeding catheter. Before any feeding is begun, the placement of the catheter in the stomach or (preferably) the small intestine must be confirmed by radiograph, as well as by auscultation and syringe aspiration. Radiography is the only certain method of determining tube position and should be repeated following any episode of severe coughing or vomiting. (Even a well-placed tube tip can be dislodged by such events.) If intermittent feedings are given, the residual is checked before each bolus, which is withheld if more than 150 ml are recovered. If nutrient is infused continuously, the residual should be checked at least twice daily and the infusion slowed if more than 150 ml are recovered. Patients who are receiving tube feedings and those with a large NG tube in place that is not draining the stomach should be maintained in the 30° (or greater) head-up position. Such patients should not be placed supine, since gastric contents reflux more easily in that position.

If a patient is at great risk for (or in the process of) vomiting, position the patient on either side and elevate the foot of the bed. In these lateral positions the glottic opening will be the most dependent part of the central airway.

Unconscious patients who are unable to protect the airway (loss of gag reflex) should be intubated with a cuffed tube. Cuffed tubes protect reasonably well against high-volume aspiration. The likelihood of significant aspiration is small when such a tube is in place and tube feeding is continuous. Nursing personnel must remain alert to the fact that the inflation channel of the cuff resembles the feeding tube lumen. Inadvertent connection of an infusion pump to the cuff lumen can have obvious adverse consequences.

Many physicians administer cimetidine, ranitidine, or antacids to patients under intensive care whose stomachs are not decompressed continually. In this way the risks of low-pH aspiration and ulceration are minimized. Tube feeding alone helps to prevent ulceration but does not reliably buffer gastric acid.

Treatment

The treatment of most food or liquid aspiration is support and prophylaxis. If massive aspiration is observed, the trachea should be suctioned immediately and oxygen administered. Corticosteroids are not of proven benefit after aspiration has occurred, unless concomitant bronchospasm fails to respond to usual bronchodilators. In the majority of acidic gastric aspirations the stomach contents are sterile, but inflammation predisposes to later bacterial superinfection. In general, it is better to wait for fever, sputum purulence, and infiltrate to develop before starting antibiotics.

Bronchoscopic lavage does little to improve acid or alkali injury because pH is rapidly neutralized by proteinaceous exudate. Lavage of particulate material from the tracheobronchial tree is highly controversial therapy. It is probably better to encourage clearance by coughing, bronchodilator therapy, and chest percussion.

If documented, chronic aspiration of gastric contents should be opposed by antireflux maneuvers. Surgical correction of a hiatal hernia may be curative. Laryngectomy and a variety of diverting or closure procedures for the larynx have been devised for intractable chronic problems due to blatant incompetence of the laryngeal sphincter. Some of these are potentially reversible if the underlying condition improves.

SUGGESTED READINGS

1. Bartlett JG, Gorbach SL. The triple threat of aspiration pneumonia. Chest 1975;68:560–66.

2. Cataldi-Betcher EL, et al. Complications occurring during enteral nutrition support: a prospective study. JPEN 1983;7:546–52.

3.   Heimlich HJ. A life-saving maneuver to prevent food choking. JAMA 1975;234:398-401.

4.   Heymsfield SB, et al. Enteral nutritional support. Metabolic, cardiovascular and pulmonary interrelations. Clin. Chest Med. 1986;7:41-67.

5.   Johanson WG, Harris GD. Aspiration pneumonia, anaerobic infections and lung abscess. Med. Clin. North Am. 1980;64:385-94.

6.   Torrington KG, Bowman MA. Fatal hydrothorax and empyema complicating a malpositioned nasogastric tube. Chest 1981;79:240-42.

7.   Wynne JW, Modell JH. Respiratory aspiration of stomach contents. Ann. Intern. Med. 1977;87:466-74.

Chapter 25

Chronic Cough

Cough is a primary defense mechanism, designed to clear the airway of irritating debris. It presents as a medical problem both when too ineffective to prevent secretion retention and when so continually active as to disrupt normal daily activity. When cough is indicated for secretion clearance, endotracheal suctioning is a poor substitute. Failure to clear the airway of secretions may result in marked airflow obstruction, especially when the airway caliber is already narrow. Atelectasis and infection are other consequences.

Three parts comprise the cough maneuver: deep inspiration, glottic closure with gas compression, and glottic release with gas expulsion. The effectiveness of cough depends upon gas flowing at high velocity in the airways.

Ineffectual Cough

The major mechanisms by which cough efficacy can be disrupted are interference with glottic closure (preventing intrathoracic pressure from building), ineffective expiratory muscle action (due to weakness or pain), and airflow obstruction. Facilitation of cough is therefore directed at these primary defects.

Glottic closure

The two primary means by which glottic function can be improved are to improve mental status and to remove any endotracheal tube that stents open the larynx. Removal of a nasogastric tube can also be helpful in re-establishing coordinated glottic closure.

Expiratory muscle action

The expiratory muscles often respond to relief of pain that otherwise prevents attainment of high lung volumes or coordinated contraction. Nutritional support, abdominal splinting or binding, and the assumption of the upright posture all promote forceful expulsive maneuvers. Chronically weakened patients may benefit from muscle training techniques.

Airflow obstruction

Relief of bronchospasm, improved secretion clearance with chest physiotherapy techniques, and the use of the upright position all help to keep airways at optimal caliber.

Persistent Cough

A chronic cough unassociated with obvious pathology is a very frequent clinical complaint. The cough reflex can be triggered at any level of the airway and can be a harbinger of serious underlying illness. More commonly, however, cough is a troublesome symptom, associated with definable and usually treatable minor pathology.

Common Etiologies of Persistent Cough

Infection and postinfection state	Nasal and sinus congestion
Neoplasia	Swallowing disorders
Obstructive lung disease	Asthma equivalent
Cardiac disease	Esophageal reflux/aspiration
Infiltrative lung disease	ENT disorder
Irritant inhalation (smoke)	Nervous tic

In otherwise healthy persons the major etiologies are postinfective, sinobronchial disease, esophageal reflux, and occult asthma.

Evaluation

History taking should focus on several high-yield areas: symptomatology suggestive of asthma, congestive heart failure, sinobronchial syndrome, nasal congestion, heartburn, episodic or exertional dyspnea, and the relation of symptoms to recumbency and sleep. A history of occupational exposure to dust and fumes or recent bronchopulmonary infection may be sufficient to allow a presumptive diagnosis. The presence of blood or blood streaking in the sputum, recent weight loss, and hoarseness are of obvious importance. Substernal chest discomfort may indicate ongoing bronchitis. A detailed physical examination must be conducted, especially of the supradiaphragmatic structures. Particular attention should be given to the ear canals and tympanic membranes, nasal mucosa and retropharynx, sinuses, lungs, and heart. The patient must be observed both upright and recumbent. A chest radiograph, electrocardiogram, and, in troublesome cases, spirometric testing are indicated. Studies directed at the swallowing mechanism, the sinuses, and the upper GI tract may be needed, as the history directs. The question of reflux/aspiration may be approached with radiographic contrast studies as well as with a radionuclide swallow and lung scan. Whereas indirect laryngoscopy is a simple office procedure that should be considered as part of the initial evaluation in most cases, fiberoptic bronchoscopy should generally be reserved for cases in which there is a history, physical finding, or radiographic indication to proceed. Patients refractory to a therapeutic trial aimed at the presumptive diagnosis are also candidates for this procedure.

Management

Whenever possible, therapy should be diagnosis specific. For example, decongestants, topical nasal steroids, or cromolyn should be prescribed for chronic nasal congestion with an allergic overtone. As a general rule, a cough that has its origin in sinus drainage is unlikely to respond until the sinus inflammation (as well as the bronchial inflammation) has cleared. Secretion purulence requires a course of antibiotics directed against the responsible pathogen. When asthma is a primary consideration a bronchodilator regimen is appropriate. In this setting, a short course of oral corticosteroids may also be effective. Reflux symptomatology demands an antireflux regimen. A nonproductive cough of short duration and undetermined etiology will most often resolve spontaneously, given sufficient time. Cough suppression may be all that is required to break a pernicious cycle of coughing and irritation that disrupts the patient's life. Although mere lubrication of the pharynx can be helpful, antitussive "expectorants" are seldom suppressive unless they contain codeine or dextromethorphan. Truly refractory cases may require hydrocodone to effect meaningful relief.

SUGGESTED READINGS

1. Corrao WM, Braman SS, Irwin RS. Chronic cough as the sole presenting manifestation of bronchial asthma. N. Engl. J. Med. 1979;300:633-37.

2. Irwin RS, Corrao WM, Pratter MR. Chronic persistent cough in the adult: the spectrum and frequency of causes and successful outcome of specific therapy. Am. Rev. Respir. Dis. 1981;123:413-17.

3. Irwin RS, Pratter MR. Treatment of cough. Chest 1982;82:662-63.

4. Irwin RS, Rosen MJ, Braman SS. Cough - a comprehensive review. Arch. Int. Med. 1977;137:1186-91.

5. McFadden ER. Exertional dyspnea and cough as preludes to acute attacks of bronchial asthma. N. Engl. J. Med. 1975;292:555-59.

6.   Poe RH, et al. Chronic cough. Bronchoscopy or pulmonary function testing? <u>Am. Rev. Respir. Dis.</u> 1982;126:160-62.

Chapter 26

Disorders of the Ventilatory Pump

RESPIRATORY MUSCLE PHYSIOLOGY

Functional Anatomy

Ventilation is accomplished by a reciprocating pump whose cylinder is the thoracic cage and whose piston is the respiratory musculature. As outlined in Chapter 1, most tidal breathing is accomplished by active inhalation and passive deflation. The inspiratory muscle group is comprised of the diaphragm (responsible for the major portion of ventilation at all but extreme work rates) and the accessory group, primarily the external and parasternal intercostals, the scalenes, and the strap muscles of the neck. Expiratory muscle action is required for expulsive efforts (cough, sneeze, defecation), for high levels of ventilation (> 20 liters/min), and for breathing against a significant resistive load (as during an exacerbation of asthma or COPD). Because maintenance of alveolar ventilation requires a pressure gradient sufficient to overcome resistive and elastic forces, any condition that leads to the inability to generate negative intrathoracic pressure will stress the system and may lead to ventilatory failure. Alternatively, conditions that increase the force requirement may lead to the same outcome, even without pump impairment. Although increased work load and impaired pump function often coexist, this section will concentrate on pump disorders that involve derangements of strength, thoracic configuration, and muscular coordination.

Muscular Strength

Muscular strength depends upon the bulk of the muscle, its contractility, the integrity of its innervation, and its loading conditions. Advanced age and poor nutrition are associated with reductions in skeletal muscle mass. Inherent contractility is influenced greatly by the chemical environment. Derangements of Ca^{++}, Mg^{++}, $PO_4^=$, K^+, CO_2, pH, and perhaps Fe^{++} are particularly important to correct. The shorter the inspiratory muscle fiber and the greater the velocity of shortening, the less forceful will contraction be for any specified level of neural stimulation. The greater the "afterload" faced by the muscle (due to resistive or elastic loading), the less effectively will muscle contraction perform useful external work.

Thoracic Configuration

However well individual muscle fibers contract, geometric alignment determines how effectively the force generated accomplishes ventilation. When totally flattened, for example, the diaphragm develops tension that tends to pull the ribs inward in an expiratory action.

Muscular Coordination

In generating negative intrathoracic pressure, the inspiratory muscles normally contract synchronously to either cause inspiratory displacement directly or to stabilize regions of the rib cage or abdomen so that the inspiratory actions of complementary muscles are not wasted in expiratory motion. Therefore, a stable chest wall and coordinated muscular activity are essential to pump efficiency.

COMMON PUMP DISORDERS

Chest Wall Configuration

Massive obesity is perhaps the most common disorder of chest wall configuration. The impedance offered by the heavy chest wall effectively afterloads the muscles of inspiration. However, although the diaphragm must push against the abdominal contents, impairing diaphragmatic descent, the abdomen can act with unusual effectiveness as a fulcrum. Thus, more active rib cage displacement may compensate for the reduced caudal displacement, so that quiet breathing is little affected. Under the stress of increased ventilation requirements, however, higher tidal volumes are needed, and the elastic work of breathing may increase dramatically. With the abdominal contents thrusting against the diaphragm, the equilibrium position of the chest wall is displaced to a lower volume, so that FRC tends to fall. This is especially true in the supine position, where abdominal forces push the underside of the diaphragm cephalad. Airway calibers are commensurately reduced and resistance to breathing increases. Moreover, the tendency for hypoxemia and positional desaturation are greatly increased because the patient tends to breathe below the "closing volume" of the lung (see p. 136). Similar arguments apply to the patient with ascites. In managing the obese or ascitic patient, special attention must be paid to maintaining an upright position and to supplementing inspired O_2.

Kyphoscoliosis and ankylosing spondylitis seriously distort the other component of the thoracic shell, the rib cage. Both disorders seriously impair the inspiratory capacity, so that the deep breaths needed for exertion or coughing are compromised. FRC tends to be well preserved. Initially the problem is purely one of configuration, although later in the course the inability to ventilate and to clear secretions effectively from disadvantaged areas can lead to reduced lung compliance. Difficulty increases in proportion to the bony deformity. In scoliosis, for example, serious respiratory problems attributable to mechanical problems are seldom evident until the angle of curvature exceeds 100 degrees. Muscles that would ordinarily have an inspiratory action can be placed into a neutral or expiratory alignment by bony distortion. What's more, the chest cage becomes difficult to deform. Maintaining the airway free from infection and concentration on nutritional factors are the keystones of effective management.

Although massive pleural effusion and pneumothorax are not generally thought of as problems of chest wall configuration, in fact they both can produce dyspnea by this mechanism. For example, either may flatten or invert the ipsilateral diaphragm and drive the accessory inspiratory muscles to a hyperinflated position. In this configuration the individual muscle fibers are foreshortened and the geometry does not permit efficient inspiratory motion. Thus, a major component of the relief of dyspnea following thoracentesis or chest tube placement relates to the recovery of mechanical advantage.

Muscular Strength and Coordination

Diaphragmatic paralysis and quadriplegia represent opposing examples of regional muscular weakness. As such, both disorders present inherent problems of impaired coordination as well as loss of effective muscle bulk and strength. A paralyzed diaphragm tends to rise rather than fall during the inspiratory half cycle. As a passive membrane, it moves in accordance with the transmural pressure gradient across it. As intra-abdominal pressure rises and intrathoracic pressure falls, the structure tends to advance into the chest.

Unilateral diaphragmatic paralysis causes only a modest impediment to ventilatory capability, with VC falling approximately 1/3 from its normal value. Quiet tidal breathing is little affected. Symptoms only surface under periods of stress or in the presence of a comorbid problem. Although causes of unilateral paralysis can sometimes by identified (e.g., tumor, infection, surgery), many such cases are idiopathic. Bilateral diaphragmatic paralysis is a devastating illness that, like its unilateral counterpart, is also usually idiopathic. These patients must sustain the entire ventilatory burden with the accessory muscles. When upright the expiratory muscles can contract to drive the diaphragm high into the chest at end expiration. When expiratory tone is released, the abdomen sucks the diaphragm down to a lower position, thus aiding inspiration. In the supine position this mechanism cannot work. Therefore these patients have extreme orthopnea and often present with sleep disturbances and headache related to CO_2 accumulation. Many such patients can sustain ventilation for many hours when upright but need periodic ventilatory support, especially at night. Although a positive-pressure ventilator is most commonly used for this purpose, a negative-pressure bodysuit can also be employed, without need for tracheostomy. Poor regional ventilation in dependent areas, frequently combined with the need for tracheostomy, causes frequent problems with atelectasis, pneumonitis, and bronchiectasis in basilar regions. Because diaphragmatic function seldom returns, treatment is supportive. Therapy centers on maintaining optimal secretion clearance, on keeping lungs free of infection, and on nutrition.

In the usual forms of quadraplegia (levels below C_5) diaphragmatic function is preserved, but the action of some of the accessory inspiratory muscles and of some or all of the expiratory group are lost. Quadriplegic patients can maintain excellent ventilation during quiet breathing but have little or no reserve. Expulsive activity is severely compromised. A pneumonia, therefore, is life threatening; secretions cannot be raised, and the ventilatory requirement is increased. Paradoxically, some quadriplegic patients breathe more easily when recumbent than when upright. Presumably, the enhanced diaphragmatic curvature of the supine position as well as the larger area of apposition of the diaphragm to the lower rib cage improves mechanical efficiency. Like diaphragmatic paralysis, the focus should center on reducing the ventilatory requirement and on keeping the lungs free of infection. When some expiratory force can be generated (thoracic cord interruptions), abdominal compression may assist the coughing effort by splinting the abdomen and allowing intrathoracic pressure to build.

SUGGESTED READINGS

1. Bergofsky EH. Respiratory insufficiency in mechanical and neuromuscular disorders of the thorax (Chapter 140). In: Fishman AP, ed. Pulmonary Diseases and Disorders. New York: McGraw-Hill, 1980;1556-66.

2. Derenne JP, Macklem PT, Roussos CH. The respiratory muscles: mechanics, control, and pathophysiology. Am. Rev. Respir. Dis. 1978;118:119-33, 373-90, 581-601.

3. Luce JM, Culver BH. Respiratory muscle function in health and disease. Chest 1982;81:82-90.

Chapter 27

Effusions and Empyema

MECHANISMS

The 1-20 ml of transudative fluid that normally lubricates the pleural surface is produced both by the parietal and visceral pleural capillaries and is reabsorbed by the parietal pleural lymphatics. The fragile mechanism maintaining a dry pleural space depends upon a delicate balance between hydrostatic and colloid osmotic forces, the integrity of the pleural membranes, and active lymphatic transport of protein. Provided that lymphatic drainage and membrane integrity are preserved, increased hydrostatic pressure in only the systemic veins (e.g., cor pulmonale) is usually insufficient to allow effusion to form; simultaneous pulmonary venous hypertension is required. Even a severe reduction in plasma oncotic pressure (albumin concentration less than 1.5 gm/100 ml) is not by itself a sufficient cause.

Because lymphatics are instrumental in removing protein from the pleural space, lymphatic congestion can cause proteinaceous effusion. Lymphatics line both thoracic and abdominal surfaces of the diaphragm and form interconnections between these sites. Fluid in the peritoneum may traverse the diaphragm either by this route or through macroscopic defects in the diaphragm.

Any disease affecting the lung that alters hydrostatic pressure, blocks lymphatics, or inflames the pleural membrane is a possible cause of effusion.

Common categories are CHF, malignancy, infection, cirrhosis, pancreatitis, pulmonary embolism (with or without infarction), lobar atelectasis, thoracoabdominal surgery, trauma, rheumatoid arthritis, Dressler's syndrome, and asbestosis.

DIAGNOSIS

Radiology

If fluid is visible on the standard upright chest film, at least 150-200 ml are present.

On a supine film, pleural fluid layers posteriorly cast a "ground glass" shadow over the affected hemithorax.

Bilateral decubitus and prone films may uncover compressed or obscured areas of the lung.

Subpulmonic effusions are common and have characteristic features (see p. 120). Drinking a carbonated beverage beforehand may aid in defining the stomach.

Unlike unilateral right-sided effusions, large unilateral left-sided effusions are very unusual in CHF and must be investigated.

Large, unilateral pleural effusions should shift the mediastinum toward the opposite hemithorax. Failure to do so suggests an immobile mediastinum or airway blockage and underlying atelectasis. Both mechanisms suggest cancer.

The weight of a massive left pleural effusion expands the chest cage and may invert the diaphragm. Both processes disadvantage the respiratory musculature and may result in marked dyspnea.

A pseudotumor is a collection of fluid, localized in a fissure, that presents as a lens-shaped opacity with tapering edges. The diagnosis is usually made by viewing a lateral film.

When a pleural effusion resolves it may organize in such a way as to entrap lung tissue at the periphery. The resulting "rounded atelectasis" may simulate a lung mass. The pathognostic "comet tail" sign is produced by the bronchovascular structures extending from the direction of the hilum to the collapsed tissue.

Diagnostic Tap

There are virtually no contraindications to careful removal of a small sample (20 ml) of pleural fluid with a syringe and 22-gauge needle. The entire procedure can be completed easily within 10 minutes and should cause minimal patient discomfort (see p. 56).

Transudate Versus Exudate

Fluid overload, CHF, cirrhosis, and nephrosis are not the only causes of "transudates." Pulmonary embolism, sarcoidosis, Meigs's syndrome, myxedema, and occasionally other normally exudative processes can generate a transudative effusion. Conversely, long-standing CHF can produce an apparently exudative effusion, especially if lymphatics are grossly congested. Currently, any one of the following findings are accepted as respresenting exudate in an atraumatically obtained specimen:

Protein: 0.5 x serum value, or 3.5 gm/dl
LDH: 0.6 x serum value, or 200 units/dl

LDH criteria appear somewhat more specific than protein criteria for an exudative process, perhaps in part because lymphatic congestion can raise total protein concentration.

Cell Count and Differential

Five to ten thousand RBC/mm^3 are necessary to tint the fluid red, but this number of erythrocytes can be recovered in an exudate of any cause.

Counts greater than 100,000 RBC/mm^3 are generally due to bleeding, infarction, or carcinoma. Rarely, CHF alone will do this. Unmistakably hemorrhagic fluids are rare in tuberculosis. Patients receiving indomethacin, aspirin, or warfarin may have bloody effusions with otherwise routine pleurisy.

Transudates tend to have low WBC counts, generally 1,500 or less. A WBC count less than 25,000 has limited diagnostic value. In the setting of a parapneumonic effusion, a WBC count greater than 25,000 suggests an infected fluid.

True empyemas are opaque and viscid. Chylous (triglyceride-containing) and pseudochylous (cholesterol-containing) fluids can mimic the turbidity of empyema.

The vast majority of fluids with lymphocytic predominance are of tuberculous or malignant origin. Conversely, either polys or lymphocytes can predominate in a tuberculous or neoplastic fluid.

Eosinophilia generally indicates long-standing air or blood in the pleural space but can signify an allergic phenomenon. Eosinophils are rarely prominent in tuberculous effusions.

Cytology

Greater than 5% mesothelial cells (recognized by a higher cytoplasm to nucleus ratio than malignant cells) suggests a diagnosis other than TB.

Approximately 2/3 of cases in which tumor causes effusion can be diagnosed if a large sample is analyzed by an experienced cytologist.

Other Determinations

Glucose

Low glucose levels occur in fluids caused by bacteria, tuberculosis, and carcinoma. A very low glucose level is characteristic of rheumatoid effusion.

Any long-standing exudative effusion with a thickened pleural peel can have a reduced glucose content because of impaired diffusion of glucose into the fluid.

Amylase

Pancreatic amylase can enter the pleural space transdiaphragmatically. Salivary amylase enters via an esophageal rupture. Occasionally, lung cancer produces a salivary variant. Amylase concentration exceeds the plasma level in all of these circumstances.

Fats and Cholesterol

Chylothorax occurs due to traumatic rupture of the thoracic duct or malignant compression of major lymphatic channels, often by lymphoma.

Trauma below the 8th thoracic vertebra causes right-sided chylothorax; trauma above that level produces a left-sided chylous effusion.

Chylous effusions are lymphocytic and contain at least 400 mg/dl of fat, which stains positive with Sudan III.

Pseudochylous (cholesterol-rich) turbid fluid is formed in long-standing inflammatory effusions (TB, RA, etc.).

pH

The exact significance of pH remains unclear. Because pleural fluid contains few protein buffers, the specimen must be drawn anaerobically, iced immediately to stop cellular metabolism, and prevented from exposure to air. A minimum of heparin should wet the barrel of the syringe.

Because low pH is believed to be the result of glucose metabolism via the anaerobic pathway, this finding can occur in any fluid with either a high count of metabolically active leukocytes or limited access to glucose (e.g., thick pleural rind). The levels of pH and glucose usually parallel one another and serve as "cross-checks." pH is virtually always very low in frank empyema. pH < 7.0 suggests that empyema will develop in a parapneumonic effusion, even when culture and Gram stain are negative (see p. 246).

High pH (> 7.40) suggests that tuberculosis is an unlikely cause.

DIAGNOSTIC WORKUP

With rare exception, large effusions should be sampled, at least once.

An exudative effusion should be investigated by pleural biopsy if tuberculosis or malignancy remains a viable undiagnosed alternative.

Ultrasonography and CT scan may be exceedingly helpful in documenting the presence of a loculated effusion and in guiding the aspirating needle.

MANAGEMENT

Large pleural effusions should be tapped to relieve symptoms, if dyspnea is not rapidly improved by other therapy. Transudates due to CHF will usually respond to diuresis, but relatively slowly. Removal of a small amount of fluid can relieve pressure against the mediastinum, improve diaphragmatic functioning, and aerate compressed parenchyma.

Pressure within the pleural space can build to high levels at the bases, due in part to the weight of the pleural fluid. "Tension hydrothorax," like tension pneumothorax, can occur with massive effusions that compress the great vessels of the mediastinum, compromise forward output, and impair the efficiency of the ventilatory musculature. Removal of several hundred ml of fluid may suffice to restore adequate respiratory and cardiovascular function.

Pleural effusions do not themselves require a tap to dryness unless symptomatic or infected. Very large collections of proteinaceous fluid or blood should be drained because of the risk of fibrotic pleural changes and permanent lung restriction.

Recurrent malignant effusions can often be controlled by pleural sclerosis via thoracostomy tube (Chapter 12).

Empyemas and some parapneumonic effusions must be drained by surgical methods (see p. 247).

SUGGESTED READINGS

1. Black LF. The pleural space and pleural fluid. Mayo Clin. Proc. 1972;47:493-506.

2. Hanke R, Kretschmor R. Round atelectasis. Sem. Roentgenol. 1980;15:174-82.

3. Light RW. Pleural Diseases. Philadelphia: Lea and Febiger, 1983.

4. Light RW, et al. Parapneumonic effusions. Am. J. Med. 1980;69:507-12.

5. Light RW, et al. Pleural effusions: the diagnostic separation of transudates and exudates. Ann. Int. Med. 1972;77:507-13.

6. Lowell JR. Pleural Effusions: A Comprehensive Review. Baltimore: University Park Press, 1977.

7. Potts DE, Levin DC, Sahn SA. Pleural fluid pH in parapneumonic effusions. Chest 1976;70:328-31.

8. Sahn SA. Pleural manifestations of pulmonary disease. Hospital Practice 1981(March):73-89.

9. Vix V. Roentgenographic recognition of pleural effusion. JAMA 1976;229:695-98.

Chapter 28

Embolism

DEFINITIONS AND MECHANISMS

Pulmonary embolism can occur with any insoluble substance that gains access to the systemic veins. Because blood filtering is a natural function of the lung, small asymptomatic pulmonary emboli may occur periodically, even in healthy persons. Distinctive syndromes have been described for embolism of air, oil, fat, tumor cells, amniotic fluid, foreign objects, and injected particulates, as well as for bland and infected fibrin clots.

Oils or fat (e.g., embolism during lymphangiography or trauma to large bones) do not impede blood flow. Rather, symptoms develop because the fatty acid products of lipid digestion produce vascular injury, capillary leak, and edema (ARDS). Steroids may help reduce the injury, but heparin is contra-indicated. Treatment is supportive.

Similarly, the major threat to life in septic embolism is not linked to the degree of vascular obstruction. Small friable fragments of infected material embolize to cause fever, toxicity, and a characteristic radiograph: multiple ill-defined infiltrates or nodules of varied sizes, with soft, irregular outlines and frequent cavitation. Perfusion defects on lung scan are, by comparison with the radiograph, unimpressive. Pelvic abscesses, infected venous catheters, septic veins, and nonsterile injections related to drug abuse are the usual primary foci. After identification, the source must be surgically isolated or removed and the infection treated vigorously with antibiotics.

Among the most frequent unanticipated but preventable causes of sudden death in hospitalized patients, bland pulmonary venous embolism is a disease that requires skillful integration of clinical and laboratory data and considerable judgment regarding the need for invasive pursuit of the diagnosis.

DIAGNOSIS

Deep Venous Thrombosis

Predisposing Factors

Stasis of blood in the venous system, injury of the vascular intima, and tendency to clot formation characterize high-risk patients. Thus, immobilization, chronic venous disease, trauma, and congestive cardiovascular or pulmonary disease are common predisposing factors.

Physical Examination

The overwhelming majority of clinically significant emboli originate in the deep veins of the pelvis and in the lower extremities, above the knees. Superficial thrombophlebitis itself poses little embolic risk but occasionally extends to the deep system.

The signs of deep venous thrombosis relate to inflammation and obstruction. Unilateral redness, heat, swelling, and pain in a lower extremity are suggestive, as are unilateral ankle and leg edema. Unfortunately, neither inflammation nor obstruction may be present or obvious, and other processes unrelated to thrombosis may cause the same findings. At least half of large vessel clots are unsuspected on physical examination.

Diagnostic Methods

Iodine-131 fibrinogen scanning is a sensitive technique for detecting the active phase of fibrinogen turnover in calf veins of nonheparinized patients. Doppler ultrasound is a flow-probing method that accurately predicts large vein obstruction when positive. It is not as sensitive as iodine-131 fibrinogen scanning in detecting nonobstructive clots. Impedence plethysmography has the same low rate of false positive results as the Doppler technique and somewhat better sensitivity. It depends upon changes in the electrical conductance characteristics of the leg as the venous system is obstructed and released. In current practice, it is perhaps the screening test with the highest yield/morbidity ratio.

Occasionally diagnostic, the radionuclide venogram is well worth doing in patients undergoing lung scan, since it can be obtained during the same injection of isotope. Sensitivity and specificity, however, are not comparable to a contrast study, especially at or below the mid-thigh level. The contrast phlebogram is simultaneously the most sensitive, definitive, time-consuming, and potentially injurious method for defining clots of the deep venous system. Unfortunately, a negative phlebogram neither assures that further emboli are unlikely nor guarantees that an intraluminal clot did not break free or re-canalize prior to the study. It is most useful in separating large vessel occlusion from cellulitis or other causes of swelling and inflammation in the extremities.

Pulmonary Embolism

Symptoms and Physical Findings

No symptom or physical finding is either universal or specific. The symptoms of embolism resolve rapidly in the first few days after the event. Signs disappear more slowly. In the urokinase cooperative trial of patients with massive and submassive emboli, the following were observed: dyspnea and tachypnea (90%); pleuritic pain (70%); apprehension, rales, and cough (50%); and hemoptysis (30%). Tachycardia (greater than 100/min) and fever occurred in a minority of cases.

Pleural pain (and infarction) is most likely to be caused by emboli of moderate size. Syncope is usually the result of massive embolism. Pulmonary artery pressures do not rise markedly unless:

1. The embolism is truly massive (obstructing half or more of the capillary bed).

2. The capillary bed was previously compromised.

Hence, right-sided gallop and increased P_2 correlate with massive obstruction.

Electrocardiogram

The electrocardiogram (ECG) appears to be sensitive but nonspecific. Even in patients without prior cardiopulmonary disease, the ECG is normal in only a small proportion. Nonspecific ST and/or T wave changes occur in the majority of patients.

Rhythm disturbances are unusual. Atrial fibrillation or flutter seldom occurs in patients without preexisting cardiovascular compromise. Similarly, bundle branch block is very unusual. Left and right bundles are affected equally often.

ECG evidence of acute cor pulmonale appears only in patients with the most severe vascular obstruction.

Blood Studies

Although hypoxemia is the rule, PaO_2 (corrected for the effect of hyperventilation with the alveolar gas equation) exceeds 80 mmHg in 10% or more of patients with submassive or massive embolism.

Biochemical tests, fibrinogen, and fibrin-split-product assays rarely assist in diagnosis. LDH, SGOT, and bilirubin are individually elevated in a minority of cases. In the absence of liver disease the triad, although suggestive of embolism, is both unusual and not entirely specific.

Chest X-ray (CXR)

The CXR is unchanged from the pre-event film in less than half of all patients and completely normal in a small minority.

Nonspecific findings, including consolidation, elevated hemidiaphragm, pleural effusion, and atelectasis, are frequent.

More specific features, including segmental oligemia (Westermark's sign) and Hampton's hump, are unusual.

Infiltrate may represent parenchymal hemorrhage (resolve rapidly without effusion) or infarction (resolve slowly, often accompanied by a bloody effusion).

Infarcts are always pleural based and cavitate frequently. Because of the dual blood supply to parenchyma, infarction occurs most commonly in patients with prior cardiopulmonary disease. When resolving, the infiltrate often rounds up to form a spheroid "nodule" and may cavitate.

Pleural Effusion

Effusions occur in approximately half of all cases; 1/3 are transudates and 2/3 are exudates.

A bloody effusion before anticoagulation suggests infarction.

Usual collections appear early and are unilateral. Most are small or moderate in volume.

Special Studies

Perfusion Scan

Because infiltrates change rapidly in hospitalized patients, a comparison CXR must be taken within hours before the scan. A perfectly normal perfusion lung scan effectively rules out a clinically significant embolism. However, a "low-probabililty" scan is not a normal scan; a substantial fraction of low-probability scans occur with proven disease. Conversely, perfusion defects highly suggestive for pulmonary emboli are reported in a substantial proportion of angiogram-negative patients.

Criteria for calling scans high probability (positive) or low probability (negative) vary with the interpreter. Experts often disagree among themselves. Consequently, the false positive rate may be very high in some centers.

Emboli isolated to the upper lobes are unusual in ambulatory patients, whose blood flow when upright distributes preferentially to the bases. Bedridden patients often violate this rule. Likewise, solitary unilateral defects due to emboli occur infrequently.

A perfusion defect much larger than a radiographic density in the same area suggests embolism; a defect the same size or smaller than the radiographic abnormality suggests that embolism is unlikely. A similar rule applies even more strongly to areas of ventilation-perfusion mismatching.

Ventilation Scan

Addition of a ventilation scan improves specificity for emboli, but matching can occur even in embolic disease as a result of bronchoconstriction, atelectasis, or secretion retention. Conversely, apparent mismatching can result when no embolus is present. Nonetheless, recent reports suggest that the pattern of V̇/Q̇ mismatching may allow a diagnosis to be made confidently.

Angiography

Angiography is the definitive test. With appropriate care it can be performed safely in the great majority of hemodynamically stable patients and often remains positive for long periods of time after the initial event. Although best performed quickly, it is worth considering within the first week after presentation. Criteria for a positive diagnosis must include an intraluminal filling defect or an abrupt "cut-off." (Oligemia or tortuosity of vessels is inadequate.) A negative angiogram, carefully done within 48 hours of the onset of symptoms, indicates a negligible risk of clinically significant embolization for weeks afterward.

The lung scan guides the selective angiographic injections. Angiograms done without selective injections, multiple views, and magnification miss a substantial fraction of small emboli. However, the clinical significance of such emboli is unclear.

DIAGNOSTIC WORKUP

Because of the complexity of making the diagnosis, no universally applicable diagnostic protocol can be recommended. It is generally agreed that a negative angiogram rules out significant risk of embolism and that a normal perfusion scan rules out the need for angiography. Between these limits, the decision to perform or withhold angiography is based in large part upon the need for diagnostic certainty. Many clinicians use the perfusion lung scan only for its value in excluding embolism or as an indication for selective angiography. Others rely heavily on patterns of scan defects for guidance. Based upon currently available information, the following strategy seems defensible:

Angiogram Definitely Needed

1. High risk for anticoagulation (CNS trauma, active peptic ulcer, etc.)
2. Thrombolytic therapy or surgical intervention contemplated
3. Parenchymal disease renders nuclear scans uninterpretable
4. Paradoxical embolism suspected

Angiogram Not Needed

Embolism Unlikely

1. Normal perfusion scan
2. Perfusion defect much smaller than radiographic abnormality
3. Ventilation defect much larger than perfusion defect

Embolism Likely

1. Multiple lobar-size or larger defects on perfusion scan and suggestive clinical history

2. $\dot{V}/\dot{Q}$ scan shows 1 or more lobar or 2 or more segmental $\dot{V}/\dot{Q}$ mismatch defects, together with a suggestive clinical history and a CXR that shows no extensive infiltrate in the involved areas

With less convincing data, the decision to perform angiography should be based on the height of clinical suspicion, the consequences of an undiagnosed embolic syndrome in patients with limited cardiopulmonary reserve, and the ability of the patient to safely undergo the procedure.

MANAGEMENT

Prognosis and Rate of Resolution

A small percentage of patients die of massive embolism before the diagnosis is made, usually within the first hour. A patient adequately anticoagulated with heparin who survives two hours or more has an excellent prognosis. If heparin is not begun, further clinically significant embolization occurs in at least 30% of cases. This number falls to less than 5% on adequate therapy, and most of those episodes occur within the first several days of treatment. Hemodynamic abnormalities usually reverse rapidly in patients who survive long enough to begin treatment, due to relocation or breakup of clot. Angiographic findings can resolve during the first 12 hours but usually require 2-3 weeks or longer for complete resolution. Scan defects also may disappear quickly, but most resolve over weeks to months. Any perfusion defect persisting after three months is likely to be permanent.

Chronic cor pulmonale due to multiple "silent" emboli rarely occurs; however, repetition of symptomatic embolic episodes can cause this problem. Furthermore, in a small percentage of cases, clot organizes within central vessels to produce a potentially treatable form of pulmonary hypertension.

Therapy

Anticoagulation

Heparin is the drug of choice, given initially by a large loading bolus (20,000 units) and subsequent continuous infusion begun 1-2 hours afterward (1,000 u/hour). Effective heparin therapy can also be given subcutaneously if necessary (7,500 units q 6 h). It is better to err on the side of overcoagulation than undertreatment in the acute period. Therefore, it is important to ensure that anticoagulation has been achieved within a few hours of starting the maintenance infusion. Heparin should not be withheld pending the results of other studies, unless the risk of anticoagulation outweighs the clinical suspicion. Because heparin catabolism varies considerably among different patients and over time in any given individual, the rate of heparin administration should be readjusted to maintain the partial thromboplastin time (PTT) about twice normal. The great majority of heparin failures (re-embolization) occur in patients who have not been kept well anticoagulated. Duration of heparin infusion should be approximately 10 days - sufficient time to allow fresh clot to dissolve or organize. The patient should be prevented from ambulating for the first 5-7 days of therapy to avoid dislodging nonadherent clots. The prothrombin time should be "in range" 1-3 days before heparin is stopped. Patients not believed to have an ongoing risk factor should receive minidose heparin until fully ambulatory.

Duration of anticoagulation should reflect the risk for recurrence. Because the risk of recurrence falls hyperbolically with time from discharge, an arbitrary duration of 3-6 months appears reasonable in patients recovering from trauma or surgery. Patients at continued high risk of recurrence, including those who have had two or more episodes, should be anticoagulated indefinitely, or until the risk abates. Although a bit more effective than fixed low doses of subcutaneous heparin, outpatient warfarin (Coumadin) requires surveillance of the prothrombin time and is associated with a higher incidence of bleeding complications.

Thrombolytic Therapy

There is no question that streptokinase accelerates the rate of clot resolution. However, it has not been convincingly shown to decrease either morbidity or mortality resulting from pulmonary embolism, while the incidence of adverse bleeding is considerably increased. For these reasons many physicians question whether there is any valid indication for these agents in venous thromboembolic disease. Although thrombolytics accelerate the resolution of venous clots, it seems reasonable to reserve these drugs for use in patients with angiographically proven massive pulmonary embolism and unstable hemodynamics. Contraindications are numerous and include any condition that predisposes to serious bleeding. Puncture of noncompressible venous sites (e.g., subclavian) must not be performed while thrombolytics are administered. These drugs are begun as soon as possible after the thrombotic event has been proven, using a loading dose and continuous volumetric (pump) infusion over a 12-72 hour period, depending upon the clinical response. Ideally, the infusion rate is altered to keep thrombin time or euglobulin lysis time between 2-5 times the control value. Protime and PTT are also prolonged. At the conclusion of therapy heparin is begun, as thrombin time and PTT fall to twice normal. Aminocaproic acid can be used topically to stop local oozing or systemically to counteract thrombolytic therapy, if serious bleeding occurs.

Surgery: Caval Interruption and Embolectomy

Surgical interruption of the vena cava should be considered for those patients who 1) sustain recurrent life-threatening emboli from the lower extremities or pelvis despite adequate anticoagulation with heparin, 2) cannot receive heparin safely, 3) suffer massive embolism and paradoxical systemic emboli, and 4) develop septic embolism from the lower extremities.

Recurrent emboli during the first few days of heparin infusion may be due to the original clot and do not necessarily indicate that heparin is ineffective. To be called a heparin failure, embolism must recur with the PTT or recalcification time held continuously in the therapeutic range over several days.

Options for interruption of the inferior vena cava include ligation, narrowing the caval lumen by clipping, and percutaneous placement of an umbrella or Greenfield filter. The clipped or umbrella-filtered vena cava clots off eventually in 1/3 or more of cases within the first two years. Large collaterals develop, through which emboli of significant size can occur.

Ligation of the vena cava forces the collateralizing process earlier and usually results in pedal edema (less of a problem with the other procedures). In experienced hands the Greenfield filter may have a significant advantage over open procedures and other inserted appliances. Reported rates of clotting are lower and efficacy greater than with alternative techniques.

Each of these methods effectively stops life-threatening embolism for at least several months. Large collaterals may develop, but most published surgical reports suggest that the risk of clinically important embolization through these vessels is low. Because venous return is impeded for a few days after caval ligation, the procedure itself can be dangerous in patients with impaired cardiac function. Caval clipping and filter insertion are better tolerated than ligation and just as effective, except in treating septic embolism.

Emergency pulmonary embolectomy is a highly morbid procedure that has few valid indications. Most patients surviving long enough for the diagnosis to be made angiographically will respond to thrombolytic or anticoagulant therapy alone. It is only in those patients who are gravely ill and deteriorating under treatment that this heroic form of therapy should be considered. On the other hand, a surgical approach to chronic recurrent embolization and pulmonary hypertension may offer the only chance of relieving disability and potentially lethal pulmonary hypertension in carefully selected individuals.

Prophylaxis

Subcutaneous ("minidose") heparin (5000 USP units q 12 h) is of proven benefit in general surgery patients. Those recovering from hip or prostatic surgery do not appear to benefit, however. Other patients at high risk for embolism may benefit, but the data are less convincing. Bedridden patients with multiple positive risk factors (obesity, myocardial infarction, peripheral edema) are appropriate candidates. Subcutaneous heparin causes symptomatic thrombocytopenia in a small fraction of patients. Other agents, such as aspirin and dipyridamole, have not been shown to be effective.

Elastic stockings and foot elevation make sense theoretically but have not shown prophylactic value in controlled trials. More active measures, such as footboards and pneumatic compression of calf muscles, appear to be effective in preventing thrombosis, but their utility in preventing embolism from larger vessels is questionable. Nonetheless, they represent an attractive alternative for patients in whom anticoagulation is ineffective. Before application of a compressive device for prophylaxis, ongoing clotting must be ruled out.

SUGGESTED READINGS

1. Bell WR, Simon TL, DeMets DL. The clinical features of submassive and massive pulmonary emboli. Am. J. Med. 1977;62:355-60.

2. Hull R, et al. Pulmonary angiography, ventilation lung scanning and venography for clinically suspected pulmonary embolism in the abnormal perfusion scan. Ann. Int. Med. 1983;98:891-99.

3. MacMillan JC, Milstein SH, Samson PC. Clinical spectrum of septic pulmonary embolism and infarction. J. Thorac. Cardiovasc. Surg. 1978;75:670-79.

4. Moser KM, Fedullo PF. Venous thromboembolism. Three simple decisions. Chest 1983;83:117-21, 256-60.

5. Sharma GV, et al. Thrombolytic therapy. N. Engl. J. Med. 1982;306:1268-76.

Chapter 29

Hemoptysis

DIAGNOSIS

Hemoptysis is the coughing of blood in gross amounts or fine streaks from a source below the glottis. Blood may appear in expectorated material but originate elsewhere. As opposed to hematemesis, fresh blood originating in the respiratory tract is always bright red, frothy, and alkaline. Furthermore, traces of blood persist in the sputum for a protracted period after initial discovery.

Light streaking of the sputum is common during exacerbations of bronchitis but subsides as the inflammation and coughing comes under control. The simultaneous use of anti-inflammatory drugs increases the incidence of hemoptysis. A prompt and full workup is indicated in the absence of ongoing bronchial inflammation, if an infiltrate is present, or if the chest x-ray remains clear but streaking does not cease with therapy.

Copious bleeding must always be investigated promptly. The correct time for bronchoscopy is during a period of active bleeding. Common causes include bronchiectasis, bronchitis, lung carcinoma, active tuberculosis, and lung abscess. In mild cases of apparently obvious origin (e.g., pulmonary infarction due to embolism), bronchoscopy may be deferred until therapy is completed and waived in favor of close follow-up if hemoptysis ceases.

Aspirated blood produces a "ground glass" appearance on the chest x-ray that clears within hours to days. The appearance of the x-ray is not reliable in determining the site of origin; blood may drain or be aspirated into the contralateral lung. Cavitary lesions in conjunction with hemoptysis should suggest squamous or large cell carcinoma, pulmonary infarction, tuberculosis, lung abscess, Wegener's granulomatosis, and aspergilloma in a preexisting bulla or cavity.

Given a stimulus to cough, impaired blood coagulation can accentuate the tendency toward hemoptysis. Anticoagulated patients and those taking aspirin are obviously predisposed to bleed. Increased capillary fragility occurs just before menses.

Diagnostic Workup

Careful ENT examination, including laryngoscopy
Chest x-ray
CBC, platelet, and coagulation studies
Gross and microscopic examination of sputum for quantity, character, presence of organisms (bacteria, TB, fungi), and cells (cytology, hemosiderin-laden macrophages)
Arterial blood gases
Bronchoscopy
Other procedures as indicated by clinical suspicion (e.g., angiography)

MANAGEMENT

Submassive Hemoptysis

No therapy is required for patients who have small amounts of blood in the sputum, other than that directed toward the primary disease.

Expectoration of larger amounts of blood (more than 30-60 ml/24 hours) should be treated by bed rest and cough suppression, without heavy sedation, if possible. Codeine is the preferred drug for this purpose. Anticoagulants and any platelet-inhibiting medications are stopped. Chest percussion is contraindicated. Patients who are not fully alert should be nursed in the lateral decubitus position with the bleeding site dependent to help avert aspiration into the opposite lung. If the bleeding site is unknown, it must be identified. This will facilitate the decision for emergent surgical intervention if unexpectedly required.

Massive Hemoptysis

The real danger of massive hemoptysis is asphyxia, not blood loss. Truly massive bleeding rarely ceases spontaneously and often recurs. Cases treated medically have a high associated mortality. On the basis of these considerations it has been argued cogently that all patients with more than 400 ml of expectorated blood in the first three hours of observation and those who expectorate more than 600 ml of blood within 24 hours should proceed to resective surgery or bronchial artery embolization, preferably after tamponade of the bleeding lesion at bronchoscopy. However, provided that the patient is stable and the expectorated volume appears to be diminishing with a conservative approach, immediate action is not necessarily required.

The bleeding site must be expeditiously identified by bronchoscopy. A straight bronchoscope can be used to pack the bleeding bronchus (if it can be identified) or to isolate the bleeding site by inflation of a Fogarty embolectomy catheter, in preparation for surgery. Fiberoptic bronchoscopy through an endotracheal tube is also feasible and can also be used to guide an occlusive catheter into position (see p. 103). Poor visibility is often limiting, however. In this setting, fiberoptic procedures should always be attempted through a wide-lumen endotracheal tube. In patients at prohibitive risk for thoracotomy, the catheter can be left in place for days - a technique that may be lifesaving. As an alternative to balloon occlusion or packing, insertion of a double lumen-tube (Robertshaw, Bronchocath, Carlens) will allow isolation and separate ventilation of each lung. In an emergency a fiberoptic bronchoscope also can be used to direct a small-diameter endotracheal tube into the main bronchus contralateral to the bleeding lung.

Although resective surgery is the definitive treatment for refractory, life-threatening hemoptysis, in many cases hemostasis can also be achieved by bronchial artery catheterization and embolization. Although effective, this technique requires a skilled angiographer and risks transverse myelitis, as the bronchial and spiral arteries exit the aorta in close proximity. In most centers it is the approach of choice only when surgery is contraindicated or declined.

SUGGESTED READINGS

1. Adelman M. Cryptogenic hemoptysis. Ann. Int. Med. 1985;102:829-34.

2. Bookstein JJ, et al. The role of bronchial arteriography and therapeutic embolization in hemoptysis. Chest 1977;72:658-66.

3. Gong H, Salvatierra C. Clinical efficacy of early and delayed fiberoptic bronchoscopy in patients with hemoptysis. Am. Rev. Respir. Dis. 1981;124:221-25.

4. Jackson CV, Savage PJ, Quinn DL. Role of fiberoptic bronchoscopy in patients with hemoptysis and a normal chest roentgenogram. Chest 1985;87:142-44.

5. Selecky PA. Evaluation of hemoptysis through the bronchoscope. Chest 1978;73(Suppl):741-45.

6. Wolfe JD, Simmons DH. Hemoptysis: diagnosis and management. West. J. Med. 1977;127:383-90.

Chapter 30

Neoplasms of the Lung

SOLITARY PULMONARY NODULES

The solitary pulmonary nodule is a single, small, rounded radiodensity at the periphery of the lung, surrounded by lucent parenchyma and unassociated with contiguous atelectasis, infiltrate, or adenopathy. The proportion of newly discovered nodules that are malignant is age related. Although rare under the age of 35 years, cancer causes approximately half of all solitary nodules in middle age and the majority of those developed by the very elderly.

Diagnosis

Two crucial pieces of information must be secured if possible: old chest films and an assessment of the radiodensity of the nodule.

Old Films

The volume doubling time of most tumors is in the range of 5 weeks to 18 months. (Diameter needs to increase by only 25% to double volume.) Hence, nodules remaining unchanged over 2 years or longer should be watched, not resected. Since cancers often develop within scars, any definite growth is cause for major concern, even if the nodule appears only slightly larger than in previous years. However, it should also be noted that histoplasma granulomas (and perhaps other types) can grow slowly and not necessarily at a uniform rate.

Assessment of Radiodensity

Generalized dense calcification usually signifies a benign cause. Dense lamellated (target) calcification suggests histoplasmosis. "Popcorn" calcification indicates hamartoma. Recently, the attenuation number (density value) assigned by CT scan has been reported as helpful. A very high number, suggesting early calcification, may correlate well with benignity. However, different scanners yield different numbers, and a radiographic "phantom" density may be needed for standardization. This issue is not yet settled.

Diagnostic Workup

Many physicians promptly excise all operable solitary nodules that are not documented to be unchanged in volume over a two-year period or that do not have a pathognomonic pattern of calcification. Other practitioners require needle biopsy, bronchoscopy, cytology, whole lung or mediastinal CT studies, or confirmation of definite growth before recommending surgery. Since needle aspiration and bronchoscopy are unlikely to provide definitive proof of a nonneoplastic process, indirect methods should usually be bypassed in favor of direct excision of a growing lesion, unless there is an excellent reason not to proceed. There are, however, exceptions to this general rule. Although the granulomas of tuberculosis and histoplasmosis contain few organisms, coccy granulomas often teem with yeast forms, so that needle biopsy may be more frequently helpful in an endemic area. A percutaneous needle biopsy (or bronchoscopy with transbronchial biopsy) may also be helpful if the physician has a low suspicion of malignancy and is strongly inclined to observe the lesion for signs of a growth (e.g., in a young patient). Patient reticence to undergo surgery without documentation of cancer is another good reason to undertake these preliminary diagnostic procedures. Since a needle aspirate will recover diagnostic cells from a malignant lesion in approximately 70-80% of cases, this information can provide evidence to change the plan of therapy.

The vast majority of cancerous pulmonary nodules are primary in the lung and have not metastasized detectably to the mediastinum or to other organs at the time of discovery. Hence, unless the mediastinum is radiographically involved or the lesion exceeds 2 centimeters in size, mediastinoscopy need not be done routinely. Furthermore, a metastatic workup is not indicated unless there are suggestive physical findings, bony pain, cerebral symptoms, or hematologic, liver enzyme, or hypercalcemic abnormalities on screening blood studies. (Two possible exceptions to this guideline are 1) a peripheral oat cell cancer for which excision is planned and 2) an apparently solitary nodule in a patient with previously resected neoplasm.)

"BENIGN" TUMORS

Diagnosis

Histology and Behavior

Most of the so-called "benign" tumors of the lung have malignant characteristics, either because of location, metastatic potential, or tendency to convert spontaneously to a recognized malignant form. Bronchial adenomas are the most common type of "benign" growth with malignant potential.

Carcinoids comprise 80-90% of adenomas, and cystadenomas (also called cylindromas or cystic adenoid carcinomas) constitute the majority of the remainder. Both types of adenoma tend to occur in major bronchi, where chief symptoms relate to hemoptysis and obstruction (wheezing, dyspnea, atelectasis, pneumonitis). Bronchial carcinoids are usually nonfunctioning and rarely produce the carcinoid syndrome until metastatic to the liver (less than 5% of cases). Both oat cell carcinoma and bronchial carcinoids derive from the Kulchitsky cell, so that it is often difficult to make the separation between them on the basis of small bronchoscopic biopsy specimens.

Cystadenomas are less bulky tumors, growing submucosally in a cylindrical fashion. These "cylindromas" frequently occur at the tracheal level, invade locally, and metastasize early; hence, prognosis is considerably worse than for carcinoids.

Hamartomas characteristically appear in middle to later life and are perhaps the only truly benign lung tumor seen commonly. Unlike adenomas, they occur peripherally, rarely cause symptoms, and virtually never metastasize or undergo malignant change. Although they may occasionally demonstrate pathognomonic popcorn calcification, the majority cannot be diagnosed without thoracotomy.

Diagnostic Workup and Management

Because most benign tumors are proximal, fiberoptic bronchoscopy can usually make the diagnosis. These lesions are vascular and tend to bleed vigorously when biopsied. Nonetheless, a biopsy should be undertaken, either with a forceps approach or with the intraluminal use of the Wang needle. Mediastinoscopy is indicated whenever the lesion is in a central bronchus.

Localized bronchial adenomas must be excised, if possible. Depending on the location and size of the tumor, a lobectomy, pneumonectomy, or "sleeve resection" (excision of the involved bronchial segment with reanastamosis) may be appropriate. Symptoms resulting from bronchial obstruction by unresectable tumors can be palliated temporarily by laser surgery, cryosurgery, fulguration, or piecemeal resection through a rigid bronchoscope.

When due to a bronchial primary, the carcinoid syndrome is associated with particularly intense episodes of flushing and hypotension and may respond to alpha-adrenergic blockade, phenothiazines, or corticosteroids.

LUNG MALIGNANCY

Primary Carcinoma

There are two major determinants of therapy for primary lung cancer - cell type and anatomic stage.

Cell Types

There are four common cell types of lung malignancy: 1) epidermoid (squamous) carcinoma, 2) adenocarcinoma, 3) small cell carcinoma, and 4) large cell carcinoma. An additional "adenosquamous" category is often used for tumors with cellular characteristics of both.   Often, no specific classification can be confidently assigned, and the lesion is termed poorly differentiated or undifferentiated carcinoma.   Depending upon the classification system used, many pathologists recognize well- and poorly differentiated types of epidermoid and adenocarcinoma. "Bronchoalveolar" is a subtype of adenocarcinoma, "oat" is a subtype of small cell carcinoma, and "giant" and "clear" are subtypes of large cell carcinoma. Better differentiated epidermoid, adeno-, and occasionally small cell carcinomas can be identified from sputum cytology; the specific variants of large cell carcinoma are less often diagnosed with confidence. From a therapeutic standpoint, the primary cellular distinction to make is small cell cancer versus non-small cell cancer.

Table 30.1. Characteristic Features of Primary Lung Carcinomas.

	Location	Metastatic Pattern	Microscopy	CXR
Epidermoid	Proximal	First to local lymph nodes, later distant	Intercellular bridges Keratin	Cavitates frequently
Adeno	Distal	Early distant	Gland structures Mucin production	Cavitates rarely
Small cell	Proximal	Very early distant	Crush artifact Scant cytoplasm	Cavitates rarely
Large cell	Distal	Early distant	Nonspecific	Rapid growth Bulky Cavitates occasionally

Staging

The TNM classification system is in widespread use. This method classifies on the basis of tumor size (T), nodal involvement (N), and the presence of distant metastasis (M).

Table 30.2. TNM Classification of Lung Cancer.

Tumor

T_x	Known present, but unknown site (e.g., cytology +)
T_0	No evidence of primary tumor
T_1	$\leq$ 3.0 cm diameter beyond lobar bronchus. No extension.
T_2	> 3.0 cm diameter. If visible endobronchially, must not be within 2 cm of carina
T_3	Tumor within 2 cm of carina or extended to mediastinum, pleural space, or chest wall

Nodes

N_0	No demonstrable metastases to nodes
N_1	Peribronchial or hilar involvement only
N_2	Mediastinal node involvement

Metastases

M_x	Not assessed
M_0	No demonstrable distant metastases
M_1	Distant metastases present

Table 30.3. Staging of Primary Lung Carcinoma.

	Occult	Stage 1		Stage 2	Stage 3
T	T_x	T_1	T_2	T_2	T_3 any N or M
N	N_0	N_0 or N_1	N_0	N_1	N_2 any T or M
M	M_0	M_0	M_0	M_0	M_1 any T or N

Risk Factors

Cigarette, cigar, and pipe smoking are associated with lung cancer, in descending order of risk. Risk returns to baseline 10-13 years after cessation, reflecting the long incubation time from induction of disease to clinical detection. All types of primary lung cancer have an increased incidence in smokers, with the strongest association for small cell and epidermoid types. Exposure to aerosolized asbestos (2x normal incidence) and cigarette smoking (20x) are synergistic (80x). A higher than normal proportion of asbestos-related cancers are poorly differentiated adenocarcinomas. Parenchymal scarring (e.g., interstitial fibrosis, old tuberculosis) also predisposes to malignancy, usually adenocarcinoma or its less common variant, alveolar cell carcinoma.

Metastatic and Nonmetastatic Syndromes

Primary lung cancer locally invades the pleural space and mediastinum and metastasizes frequently to liver, bone, brain, and adrenal glands. Of the wide variety of nonmetastatic syndromes produced by lung cancer, osteoarthropathy, hypercalcemia, inappropriate ADH, and neuromuscular manifestations are the most common. Osteoarthropathy can best be confirmed by bone scan and x-rays of the affected area and treated by removal of the tumor or thoracic vagotomy. Corticosteroids are palliative. Osteoarthropathy rarely occurs with small cell cancers.

Hypercalcemia can result from release of nonmetastatic ectopic para-thormone or prostaglandin, as well as from direct bony invasion. Inappropriate ADH is most frequently associated with small cell tumors and often responds to demeclocycline (150 mg q.i.d.) Nonmetastatic neuromuscular manifestations of lung cancer include 1) the Eaton-Lambert syndrome of proximal muscle weakness, 2) cerebellar degeneration, 3) encephalopathy, 4) peripheral sensorimotor neuropathy, and 5) transverse myelitis.

Tumors Metastatic to the Thorax

Nodules

The majority of blood-borne metastases distribute to the peripheral interstitium of the lung and, hence, usually do not cause hemoptysis or obstruction. Sputum cytology is usually not helpful for the same reason. Multiple tumor nodules lack the uniform size of granulomata and are more profuse in regions of higher blood flow. They tend to have irregular outlines or lobulated margins and, with the exception of certain sarcomas, rarely calcify. If the primary source of the tumor nodules is not already known at the time of their discovery, strong clues are almost invariably present on physical exam, urinalysis, or routine blood studies. Breast, bone, renal, and lung sources are most common, but almost any type of tumor cell trapped by the capillary seive of the lung can grow there. However, macro- and microscopic tumor embolism from trophoblastic, breast, renal, and GI primaries can cause syndromes of acute or subacute cor pulmonale without actual invasion of lung tissue. Endobronchial metastases are rare but occasionally result from hypernephroma, melanoma, breast, and colonorectal sources.

Solitary metastases to the lung are most likely to originate from sarcoma, melanoma, colon, renal, head/neck, prostate, or gastric tissues. They may appear synchronously or long after the primary has been removed. Solitary lesions should be removed after a metastatic workup, unless there are other organs involved or the primary is unresectable. Second lung primaries are 10 times as frequent as in the general population, and the prognosis after resection of solitary metastases is favorable, especially if the deposit surfaces long after the primary was treated.

Lymphangitic Spread

Lymphangitic carcinoma involving the lung is most often due to primaries of the lung, breast, stomach, and pancreas. The course is inexorably downhill once lymphangitic disease appears; death usually results within weeks to months. Lymphangitic spread is detected on the chest film by Kerley-B lines, lung infiltrates, lymphadenopathy, and pleural effusion, in various combinations.

Pleural Metastases

Lung cancer may cause pleural effusion by direct invasion, hematogenous seeding, lymphatic congestion, and associated pneumonia or atelectasis. Although unusual, local invasion of the pleura and chest wall (without effusion) does not itself contraindicate an attempt at resection.

The superior sulcus or "Pancoast" tumor (caused by any of the primary cell types) often presents with chest wall, neck, or arm pain at a time when the only noticeable change on x-ray is thickening of the apical pleural stripe. Tumor implants of the pleural space can arise from virtually any malignancy. However, primaries of the breast, lung, and ovary account for the large majority.

Diagnosis

Tumors located proximally may present with a new cough, hemoptysis, or obstructive pneumonitis and dyspnea. Peripheral lesions usually achieve larger size before symptoms develop. Hemoptysis is more frequent with proximally located than with distally located neoplasms.

Changed voice, paralyzed hemidiaphragm, dysphagia, Pancoast symptoms, pleural effusions, the superior vena caval syndrome, and Horner's triad strongly suggest spread to extrapulmonary intrathoracic structures.

On physical examination careful attention should be directed to the skin, fingernail beds, supraclavicular nodes, eyelids and pupils, upper thoracic veins, and liver.

Diagnostic Workup

The purpose of the workup is twofold: 1) to determine the presence and cell type of cancer and 2) to assess resectability.

All Patients

Careful physical examination
Chest radiograph
Arterial blood gases
Hemoglobin, WBC, platelets
Chemistry battery (Na^+, Ca^+, SGOT, Alk. Phos.)

Selected Patients

Sputum Cytology (x 3)

Sputum cytology is very often positive with central lesions. However, the yield for small peripheral or metastatic lesions is sufficiently poor to make it optional in those cases.

Bronchoscopy (Chapter 17)

Fiberoptic bronchoscopy can usually make the diagnosis in cases of central lesions and help determine the feasibility of resection. Bronchoscopy will usually not make the diagnosis on small, peripheral lesions. In patients with worrisome symptoms (new cough, hemoptysis, hoarseness, etc.), bronchoscopy can evaluate the cords and make an early diagnosis of endobronchial neoplasia, even when the lesion is not visible radiographically. A transluminal (Wang) needle can be used to collect cells from the retrobronchial mediastinum. When positive, such information provides evidence of extension and nonresectability.

Needle Biopsy (Chapter 18)

Small peripheral lesions and those in areas difficult to reach with a bronchoscope (apex, superior segment, anterior segments of the upper lobes) can often be entered successfully with a transthoracic needle.

Mediastinoscopy / Sternotomy (see p. 110)

To ensure operability, mediastinal nodes of enlarged or questionable size by CT are usually sampled prior to thoracotomy. Many surgeons also perform a mediastinoscopic procedure when the primary cancer is radiographically large or centrally located. Bronchoscopy should precede mediastinal investigation because bronchoscopic findings alone often contraindicate surgery (small cell histology, tracheal or carinal invasion, positive Wang needle aspirate from the subcarinal level, etc.). On the other hand, many tumors that remain unsampled and undiagnosed by bronchoscopy can be diagnosed by these surgical techniques.

Supraclavicular Node Biopsy

Any palpable supraclavicular node should be biopsied as the first invasive procedure, because a postive result can circumvent further workup.

CT Scan (see p. 122)

A CT scan can determine chest wall or mediastinal invasion and detect other nodules not seen on routine chest films.

Metastatic Workup

As a general rule, a metastatic workup (bone, brain, and liver scans, bone marrow biopsy, etc.) should be directed by abnormal findings and reserved for patients with specific indications: hepatomegaly, transaminase elevation, bone pain, CNS symptoms, anemia, hypercalcemia, etc. Exceptions to this rule occur when resection of a peripheral oat cell carcinoma or apparently "solitary" pulmonary metastasis is contemplated. Asymptomatic patients having normal physical examination, screening CBC, and chemistry battery rarely have detectable metastatic disease.

Preoperative Evaluation

The risks associated with resective surgery are those that accompany major surgery of any type and those associated with removal of lung tissue.

Risks Unrelated to Resection

Intraoperative Risk

The stresses of anesthesia, extensive surgery, and fluid resuscitation may overwhelm a marginally compensated cardiovascular system. Poorly controlled right or left heart failure, recent myocardial infarction, and symptomatic ventricular ischemia or arrhythmia present prohibitive hazards for elective procedures.

Postoperative Risk

Any patient who undergoes thoracic or abdominal surgery may develop postoperative pulmonary complications related to inadequate ventilation and defective airway clearance. Although the incidence of atelectasis, ventilatory insufficiency, and pneumonia is acceptable for lower abdominal operations, it rises dramatically for incisions made near the diaphragm, which impair cough, ventilatory mechanics, and diaphragmatic function. Patients at highest risk are those whose ability to maintain bronchial patency is impaired preoperatively by airflow limitation, excessive airway secretions, obesity, or neuromuscular weakness.

Risks Related to Resection

Two additional risks are posed by resection of lung tissue: 1) limitation of ventilatory capability and 2) induction of cor pulmonale. Both can cause perioperative death or crippling ventilatory insufficiency after recovery. The chance of death during resective surgery depends upon the severity of underlying lung disease, the presence of cardiovascular disease, the age of the patient, and the extent of the procedure. Approximately 5% of all well-selected lobectomy patients and 10% of pneumonectomy patients fail to survive the perioperative period.

Patients should not be subjected to resection if the chances of operative death or truncated survival due to ventilatory insufficiency exceed those of cure. The likelihood of 5-year survival without recurrence in good-risk operable patients ranges from 20% to 60%, depending upon tumor type, size, and proximity to the carina.

Patient Selection by Pulmonary Function Testing

Lung cancer and impaired ventilatory reserve frequently coexist because these disorders share common etiologic factors (cigarette smoking, asbestos exposure, interstitial fibrosis).

Chronic Airflow Obstruction

1) Screening Tests

Many pulmonary function tests have been reported to predict post-operative ventilatory function. Blood gas values are unreliable, since hypoxemia may originate in the abnormal lung, and $PaCO_2$ may be elevated by central insensitivity to CO_2 rather than by impaired mechanics. Exercise tests are sensitive but nonspecific. If a patient can negotiate several flights of stairs without stopping due to dyspnea or can complete the advanced stages of a formal exercise test, the likelihood of tolerating pneumonectomy is high. Failure to do so should not preclude surgery without further evaluation of the underlying cause.

Static tests of mechanics and gas exchange provide better discrimination. Patients meeting all of the following criteria generally undergo pneumonectomy without prohibitive risk:

FVC	50% of predicted
FEV $_1$	50% of FVC, or 2 liters
MVV	50% of predicted
RV/TLC	50%
D_LCO	50% of predicted

Mechanics should be optimal before spirometry is attempted.

Blood flow does not distribute evenly in patients with neoplasia; only a very small minority ($\simeq$ 5%) of patients have greater perfusion to the ipsilateral lung. Furthermore, postoperative spirometry is often far better than predicted on the basis of the tissue volume removed, especially in patients with partially occlusive tumors of the central bronchi. Hence, failure by one or more of the above criteria does not indicate inoperability without some assessment of the ventilatory work load carried by the noncancerous lung.

2) Split-Function Studies

a) Bronchospirometry Cumbersome and outmoded.

b) Radionuclide studies Empirically, postpneumonectomy FEV_1 has been demonstrated to be well predicted by multiplying preoperative FEV_1 by the fraction of total counts that distribute to the noninvolved lung. (Perfusion counts appear to correlate better than ventilation counts with postoperative function.) The explanation for this relationship is that growing cancers tend to redirect an increasing proportion of blood flow to the contralateral lung. Unfortunately, although a highly unilateral distribution makes resection feasible from a pulmonary function standpoint, it also means that metastases are likely to have occurred.

c) Lateral position test This simple test compares the increase in FRC induced by going from the supine to right lateral decubitus position with that induced by a similar maneuver to the left. It apportions function to the uppermost lung in accordance with the percentage of the total change in FRC caused by that shift. This test is reported to correlate surprisingly well with radionuclide assessment.

d) Balloon occlusion of the ipsilateral pulmonary artery Failure to achieve acceptable predicted values for lung mechanics does not necessarily contraindicate surgery if the predicted post-operative FEV_1 is only marginally less than the minimum acceptable value and pulmonary hemodynamics are permissive. However, lung resection will likely precipitate cor pulmonale, if significant pulmonary hypertension develops when all blood flow is directed to the noninvolved lung during balloon occlusion of the ipsilateral pulmonary artery.

3) Criteria Contraindicating Pneumonectomy

a) Predicted postoperative FEV_1 less than 800 ml Although arbitrary, this requirement has a physiologic and epidemiologic rationale. On an actuarial basis, the incidence of CO_2 retention increases, activities of daily living are curtailed, and the projected 5-year mortality due to airflow obstruction increases below this level of reserve. However, the stringency with which this criterion is applied should be modified in response to the patient's age, sex, and height.

b) Contralateral exercise PA pressure exceeds 35 mmHg Based on studies of acute pulmonary embolism, the nonhypertrophied right ventricle cannot sustain a mean pulmonary artery pressure greater than 35 mmHg without decompensating. Hence, a preoperative pressure approaching this level suggests that the capillary bed has already been severely restricted and will not tolerate further losses.

The validity of these criteria regarding perioperative morbidity and mortality has been adequately demonstrated. However, a study that carefully documents long-term functional outcome using these guidelines is not available.

If lobectomy rather than pneumonectomy is contemplated, all criteria (both screening and split function) can be 20-25% worse and still permit surgery.

Within broad limits, the incidence of disabling cor pulmonale in patients with COPD parallels declining ventilatory function, as measured by rates of maximal airflow. Hence, independent evaluation of the pulmonary vascular bed in these patients usually is unnecessary, unless there is a suspicion of symptomatic pulmonary hypertension or the patient fails to meet the split-function FEV_1 criteria.

Restrictive Disease

Criteria based on rates of maximum airflow are somewhat inappropriate to apply to patients with restrictive disease. Nonetheless, FVC, FEV_1, MVV, and $D_L CO$ all tend to reflect the severity of restriction, and in the absence of convincing prospective clinical studies, they are commonly applied.

Management

Surgery

With the exception of small cell carcinoma, resection is the treatment of choice. The smallest amount of lung tissue is removed that is consistent with complete excision, technical feasibility, and adequate postoperative functional reserve. For solitary metastases and small peripheral nodules, a "wedge" resection is appropriate. For larger lesions lobectomy or pneumonectomy is required.

Nonresectable conditions include

1) small cell tumors, other than peripheral nodules
2) distant metastases
3) superior vena caval obstruction
4) recurrent laryngeal nerve involvement

5) malignant cells in pleural fluid
6) contralateral lymph node metastases
7) involvement of the trachea, carina, or contralateral main bronchus
8) metastasis above the aortic arch in left mediastinum
9) metastasis to highest node group in right mediastinum

Local chest wall invasion, localized pericardial penetration, and ipsilateral intranodal involvement with epidermoid carcinoma place the patient at high risk for recurrence but are not considered absolute contraindications to resection by most surgeons.

Chemotherapy

Chemotherapy is of proven benefit only in small cell carcinoma, where combined with irradiation of the neural axis, it is the standard of therapy.

Radiation

Preoperative irradiation appears to be of benefit only in treatment of superior sulcus tumors.

Adjunctive irradiation (postresection) is often given when nodes sampled at surgery are involved by tumor. Although the small tumor burden makes this approach attractive, efficacy remains unproven.

Curative radiotherapy is a reality in a very small percentage of unresectable patients. It may be worth trying if the tumor bulk is small and the patient is otherwise inoperable.

Palliative irradiation is the primary modality for treating bony pain, the superior vena caval syndrome, intracerebral metastases, and symptomatic bronchial obstruction.

Superior Vena Caval (SVC) Syndrome

Compression of the SVC most commonly results from small cell carcinoma. Although gradual in onset, the SVC syndrome should be treated promptly once symptoms develop. If respiratory compromise occurs (due to tracheal compression and glottic edema), this problem can present a genuine emergency.

Radiotherapy requires several days to exert its beneficial effect, during which time further narrowing of airways and vessels can be anticipated due to inflammatory swelling. The following treatment approach appears justified:

Head elevated
Prednisone (20 mg q 6 h) for one day before and for three days after
  starting radiation therapy
Radiation with or without chemotherapy
Mild diuresis
Anticoagulation
Intubation tray at the bedside

SUGGESTED READINGS

1.   Boysen PG. Assessment for lung resection. Respir. Care 1984;29:506-15.

2.   Dumon JF, et al. Treatment of tracheobroncheal lesions by laser photo-resection. Chest 1982;81:278-84.

3.   Geddes DM. The natural history of lung cancer. A review based on rates of tumor growth. Br. J. Dis. Chest 1979;73:1-17.

4.   Hande KR, DesPrez RM. Current perspectives in small cell lung cancer. Chest 1984;85:669-77.

5.   Heitzman ER. Bronchogenic carcinoma. Radiologic - pathologic correlation. Semin. Roentgenol. 1977;12:165-74.

6.   Lillington G. The solitary pulmonary nodule - 1974. Am. Rev. Respir. Dis. 1974;110:699-707.

7.   Madewell JE, Feigin DS. Benign tumors of the lung. Semin. Roentgenol. 1977;12:175-86.

8.   Matthay RA. Recent advances in lung cancer (symposium). Clin. Chest Med. 1982;3:217-454.

9.   Mountain CF, Carr DT, Anderson WA. A system for the clinical staging of lung cancer. Am. J. Roentgenol. Radium Ther. Nucl. Med. 1974;210:130-38.

10. Tisi GM, et al. Clinical staging of primary lung cancer. Am. Rev. Respir. Dis. 1983;127:659-64.

Chapter 31

Pneumonic and Pleural Infections-Bacterial

PNEUMONIA

Pathogenesis

Organisms usually enter the lower respiratory tract in aspirated pharyngeal or upper airway secretions. Inhalation of an infective aerosol and hematogenous seeding are other mechanisms. Normally, effective glottic closure, cough, and mucociliary clearance provide mechanical defenses against contamination. When any of these are disrupted, pneumonitis can begin, especially if underlying host defenses are compromised. In the community, pneumococcus, mycoplasma, and legionella are common pathogens in otherwise healthy adults. Patients with chronic obstructive pulmonary disease are prone to infections with Hemophilus influenzae and Branhamella catarrhalis as well as the common organisms. Elderly adults, especially those who are debilitated or cared for in a communal facility are often colonized with Gram-negative organisms such as klebsiella/enterobacter and e. coli. Staphylococcus is also a frequent offender in this group. All too often, a specific pathogen cannot be identified despite good sampling methods and overt symptomatology compatible with an acute bacterial process. Mixed aerobic/anaerobic infection, mycoplasma, chlamydia, legionella, and viral agents are likely candidates to explain the process under these conditions.

Diagnosis

The choice of initial therapy for a bacterial process is always accompanied by some uncertainty, even in the presence of a Gram stain "typical" for a specific organism. Historical features can help immensely in sorting through the diagnostic possibilities. For example, the sudden onset of chills, pleurisy, rigors, and high temperature are characteristic features for pneumococcus in a young adult. On the other hand, these findings may be inconspicuous in an older person. Confusion or stupor often predominate in the elderly. A history of seizures, drug abuse, alcoholism, or swallowing disorder focuses attention on the possibility of aspiration. Recent travel history, occupational exposure, and concurrent family illnesses can help to make the diagnosis of an unusual etiology. The physical examination is less helpful than either the history or the chest roentgenogram. Occasionally, however, bullous disease, a skin rash, gingival disease, or purulent sinus drainage will help to narrow the differential possibilities.

Numerous classical roentgenographic features have been described, including lobar consolidation with air bronchograms (pneumococcal pneumonia), lobar consolidation without air bronchograms (central obstruction), bulging fissures (klebsiella), infiltrate with ipsilateral hilar adenopathy (histoplasmosis, tularemia, tuberculosis), widespread cavitation (staphylococcus), and sequential progression to multilobar involvement (legionella). These findings are not sufficiently consistent, however, to be of real value in confirming the diagnosis. For example, virtually any pneumonia can mimic an interstitial infiltrate, cavitation, or pneumatocele formation in a patient with emphysema.

Laboratory studies are the cornerstone of the diagnostic workup. Blood leukocyte count and differential can be of significant help. Leukopenia is often seen in overwhelming infections due to staphylococcus, pneumococcus, and klebsiella, placing the patient in a guarded prognostic category. A differential count that is not significantly left-shifted suggests the possibility of a viral, mycoplasmal, or atypical bacterial pathogen. When performed correctly, stain and culture of pulmonary secretions remains the most likely technique to yield a diagnosis. Apart from the Gram stain, coagulation tests (H. influenzae, klebsiella) and direct immunofluorescent antibody staining (legionella) are other useful methods for processing the expectorated sample that can yield an immediate, if presumptive, diagnosis. Expectorated sputum is appropriate for analysis and culture if there is a high ratio of inflammatory to epithelial cells. Inhalation of a hypotonic or hypertonic aerosol, particularly if given via an ultrasonic nebulizer, can often encourage a productive cough in patients otherwise unable or unwilling to expectorate (see p. 74). When adequate sputum cannot be obtained, nasotracheal or transtracheal catheterization (Chapter 14) can be helpful. Occasionally, more invasive methods are indicated, including bronchoscopy using the protected brush technique and/or lavage. In general, these procedures should be reserved for those who are seriously ill, immune compromised, or unresponsive to conventional therapy. Transthoracic needle aspiration often yields an adequate specimen but exposes the patient to attendant risks of pneumothorax and bleeding. Open lung biopsy should rarely be considered in patients who have intact host defenses. Cultures of the blood and pleural fluid must be obtained and, when positive, are the most convincing evidence of the responsible organism. Unfortunately, such specimens are often negative, even in seriously ill patients.

Treatment

In the hospital, nutritional, fluid, electrolyte, and oxygen support of the patient with bacterial pneumonia are noncontroversial and universally applied. The initial choice of antibiotic must be guided not only by the nature of the suspected organism but also by the severity of illness. Thus, although treatment should be directed as specifically as possible in patients who are only moderately ill, the initial therapy of a compromised patient with serious illness should include broad spectrum coverage until culture results are available. Many patients with pneumonia require adjunctive therapy. For example, a patient with severe airflow obstruction will often benefit from bronchodilator administration and chest physiotherapy techniques to help clear airway secretions.

LUNG ABSCESS

Pathogenesis

Necrotizing lung infections often result in tissue necrosis and abscess formation. Primary lung abscess accounts for about 2/3 of all lung abscesses and results from the aspiration of mixed oropharyngeal flora. Patients with primary lung abscess typically have undergone a recent loss of consciousness, e.g., from alcohol or drug intoxication, generalized seizures, or recent anesthesia for surgical or dental procedures. Periodontal disease is another important predisposition. Presentation can be one of acute febrile illness or chronic indolent wasting disease. Anaerobic organisms figure prominently in the pathogenesis of primary lung abscesses. A large inoculum of organisms can be aspirated as an infective nidus of gingival debris or sinus drainage. Alteration of lung tissue by aspirated gastrointestinal contents may also set the stage for abscess formation. Primary abscesses tend to develop in the dependent lung regions and therefore are more common in the right than the left lung and in posterior rather than anterior regions.

Radiographically, the lung abscess appears as a thick-walled, rounded infiltrate, usually with an air-fluid level if it has been in recent communication with the tracheobronchial tree. Abscess can usually be distinguished from a fluid-filled or infected bulla, in that the latter has a thin-walled upper margin. The distinction is important, because lung abscess requires more lengthy and/or aggressive antibiotic therapy. Distinction of an abscess from an empyematous bronchopleural fistula is often surprisingly difficult. The standard 2 view radiograph will generally show an air-fluid level in both. Computed tomography is often the best way to make such distinctions. An empyema is always contiguous with the chest wall and usually has either the frontal or lateral dimension significantly longer than the other. An empyema cavity often changes shape with variation in position. A lung abscess near the chest wall makes an acute angle with it, whereas an empyema produces an obtuse angle. The differential diagnosis of primary lung abscess includes empyema, necrotizing pneumonia, neoplasm, or infected bulla. Of these, necrotizing pneumonias secondary to staphylococcus, klebsiella, and other Gram-negative pneumonias are perhaps the most common.

Treatment

Virtually all primary abscesses result, at least in part, from anaerobes such as fusobacteria, bacteroides, microaerophilic streptococci, and peptostreptococci. Although the majority of these infections respond to penicillin in a dosage of $6-12 \times 10^6$ units/day, a certain fraction of bacteroides species are resistant, and clindamycin or an appropriate cephalosporin is a good choice for refractory organisms and penicillin-allergic patients. If anaerobic culture is attempted (rarely necessary), the transtracheal approach or protected catheter technique is essential to avoid oral contamination. Antibiotics should be continued until all clinical manifestations have resolved and the radiographic appearance has stabilized. In general, 4-8 weeks are required for this process. Oral therapy (penicillin at 750 mg q.i.d.) can be administered within a few days of defervescence and clinical response. If specific pathogens are identified, antibiotic management should of course be appropriately directed, following similar guidelines for duration and dosage.

Apart from antibiotic therapy, nutritional support and adequate drainage must be established. Nearly always, this spontaneously occurs. When drainage is sudden and a large cavity spills its contents into the tracheobronchial tree, an overwhelming aspiration pneumonitis can develop, resembling ARDS. This unfortunate outcome is especially likely in obtunded patients. Other untoward complications include massive hemoptysis (secondary to erosion of a large vessel) and infective seeding to intracerebral or intrapleural sites.

Bronchoscopy should be reserved for patients in whom there is a strong suspicion of an obstructing foreign body or lung tumor, for those who fail to respond to medical therapy, and for patients in whom the question of underlying tuberculosis, fungal disease, or lung cancer is sufficiently strong to warrant the procedure prior to embarking on a lengthy antibiotic regimen. The technique of attempting to open a nondraining cavity by bronchoscopic intervention risks massive aspiration, either at the time of the procedure or shortly thereafter. Such patients must be closely observed postprocedure. Surgical intervention is now needed only rarely. Generally accepted indications are massive hemoptysis, strong suspicion of tumor, and failure of a symptomatic patient to respond to antibiotics alone.

EMPYEMA

Mechanisms

Bacterial contamination of the pleural space can follow thoracic surgery, penetrating wounds of the thorax, subdiaphragmatic infection, esophageal rupture, or hematogenous seeding of sterile fluid. However, the most common etiology remains parenchymal lung infection, despite the current availability of potent antibiotics.

Radiographically detectable parapneumonic effusions are exceedingly common and result from any type of infectious pathogen. In contrast, parapneumonic empyema is distinctly uncommon and tends to occur in aged, debilitated, and alcoholic patients. Usually the result of neglected or undetected parenchymal infection, bacterial empyema rarely develops if appropriate antibiotics are given soon after the infection begins.

Diagnosis

Natural History

The natural history of empyema includes three phases. The initial exudative phase is characterized by an uncontaminated thin serous fluid that usually reabsorbs without sequelae. In those who develop empyema, the fibrinopurulent phase follows, with organisms, frank pus, and fibrin loculations. In the final organizing phase, a thick inelastic peel develops that occasionally causes symptomatic restriction of lung function. The major diagnostic problem is to separate infected from uninfected fluid.

Symptoms

Usually insidious in onset, empyema produces low-grade fever in 80% of patients. Chest pain, weight loss, productive cough, chills, dyspnea, night sweats, and tenderness of the chest wall occur in declining order of frequency. Chronic empyema may extend over months, with few symptoms other than weight loss.

Bacteriology

No pathogen is grown from many fluids infected by fastidious anaerobes, despite a positive Gram stain. If anaerobic cultures are done carefully, purely anaerobic, purely aerobic, and mixed isolates are about equally common. A single pathogen is isolated in a minority of cases; most empyemas are polymicrobial. Of community-acquired empyemas, staphylococcus, streptococcus, pneumococcus, and Hemophilus influenzae are the most frequent aerobic pathogens.   Gram-negative rods, staphylococcus, and enterococcus are the most common isolates from patients contracting their disease in a hospital. Pneumococcal empyema characteristically develops after the pneumonic process has subsided, perhaps accounting for the rarity of pneumococcal empyema since the availability of antibiotics.

Diagnostic Workup

Thoracentesis (pH and glucose, WBC, protein, LDH, Gram stain, culture for
  bacteria and tuberculosis)
CBC
Blood cultures
CXR (PA, lateral, and decubitus)
Thoracic CT Scan
Thoracic ultrasound to identify loculations of fluid
Sputum (AFB, bacterial smear and culture)

Management

Parapneumonic Effusion

It is clear that some very small infected effusions respond to antibiotics without drainage, if therapy is initiated soon after the onset of illness. However, sizable collections of infected fluid eventually progress to loculate and cause protracted illness, so that drainage of larger empyemas should be initiated without delay. Hence, parapneumonic effusions large enough to tap should be sampled as soon as discovered, If the clinical suspicion of empyema is strong (e.g., because of a continued adverse course despite antibiotics) and loculations are obvious by ultrasound, fluid should be aspirated from several sites if the first samples appear benign. Recrudescence or persistence of fever, positive culture from the initial tap, and an increase in volume of the effusion after several days of antibiotic therapy are excellent indications to resample the fluid and place a chest tube if the findings warrant.

The fluid characteristics that justify drainage by thoracostomy tube are somewhat controversial. Few would argue with the need for tube drainage of gross pus or a large collection of thin fluid with organisms on Gram stain. There is disagreement as to approach in less obvious cases. Because infected fluids characteristically have low glucose and pH as well as high protein, LDH, and leukocyte counts, fluids with these characteristics may be the result of pleural space infection, even if not obvious by microscopy.

It has been shown in experimental animals that fluids inoculated with organisms transiently develop a low pH and that pH often rises again as the infection clears without the aid of antibiotics. Hence, timing of the tap may be very important regarding the pH value. Nonetheless, many good clinicians would place a chest tube for fluid with a pH less than 7.20 (and less than 0.15 units below the pH of an arterial sample). On the basis of published data, this approach appears justified if low glucose, high LDH, and elevated leukocyte count in the fluid corroborate the impression of infection. Otherwise, tapping the collection to near dryness and repeating the tap 24 hours later to assess the directional changes in volume, pH, glucose, and leukocyte count seems a good strategy. There is a tendency for large collections of proteinaceous fluid to organize, even if not infected. Slow healing then occurs by slow reabsorption or fibrosis. Tapping to near dryness lessens this risk and allows assessment of progress to be made more easily.

Bacterial Empyema

The principles of treating established empyema are to drain the infected space and to reappose the lung to the chest wall to preserve lung function and prevent recurrence. Organism-specific systemic antibiotics are adjunctive therapy, helping to limit parenchymal infection during the early phase until open drainage is established and fever remits.

Repeated Thoracentesis

With rare exceptions, repeated thoracentesis is not sufficient to achieve complete drainage of infected fluid and only enhances the risk of loculation.

Chest Tube Thoracostomy

Continuous closed drainage by chest tube is the method of choice for most empyemas in the exudative or fibrinopurulent phases. The technique of chest tube drainage is discussed in Chapter 11. A large tube is inserted into the most dependent portion of the empyema space and attached to suction drainage. (As the fluid thickens and a peel forms, irrigation with saline, antibiotics, or enzymes may aid evacuation.) If the pleural abscess is well drained, the patient should experience defervescence within three days and subsequently remain afebrile. If not, a second tube placed into another undrained pocket (located by ultrasound or CT and thoracentesis) may achieve the desired response. An open drainage procedure may be needed.

Water-seal suction drainage should be maintained for 10-14 days, by which time a sufficient peel has formed to prevent collapse of the lung when the drain is opened to atmosphere. At that point, a contrast injection can be made to determine the extent of the residual cavity. A small cavity allows the tube to be pulled back in stages, as an irrigation and open-tube drainage program is begun.   A larger cavity must be allowed better drainage; thoracotomy with decortication or open drainage is indicated. Air-fluid levels signify inadequate drainage of the pocket.

Open Drainage

If tube thoracostomy fails or if multiple loculations and a peel are present from the outset, open drainage or decortication is required. Rib resection is performed at the most dependent portion of the empyema cavity, and the skin is sutured to the parietal pleura. Although very effective and relatively well tolerated by debilitated patients, months of irrigation and drainage may be necessary for the wound to close.

Decortication and Empyemectomy

Following adequate therapy for empyema, a thickened pleural peel may either resolve slowly over many months or trap the lung. Pleural stripping (decortication) may restore pulmonary function in patients with ongoing symptomatic restriction. Careful pulmonary function testing should precede operation. Removal of the peel and excision of the empyema pocket provides an excellent alternative for good-risk patients in whom a chronic open drainage regimen would be impractical or unacceptable (e.g., young, active people).

Thoracoplasty

Thoracoplasty is now seldom necessary. However, when the lung is fibrotic and cannot expand to fill the pleural space, additional surgical procedures, including thoracoplasty, may be needed if resection or decortication cannot be done. Because resective surgery in active tuberculosis is notoriously complicated by stump breakdown, a thoracoplasty may be especially useful in the management of tuberculous bronchopleural fistula.

Postpneumonectomy Empyema

Resection of a lung creates a void that is filled by serosanguinous fluid, providing an excellent culture medium. Inoculation of bacteria at surgery or hematogenous seeding can occur. Most infections do not involve the entire thoracic cavity and may be surprisingly indolent, surfacing months to years after contamination. Dependent, open-window drainage should be established in most cases, with irrigations daily for 4-8 weeks. At that time debridement, instillation of antibiotic solution, and definitive closure has been a successful strategy.

Bronchopleural Fistula

An open communication between the airway and pleural space should be suspected if the patient continues to expectorate large amounts of purulent sputum, especially when placed in a lateral decubitus position. Air-fluid levels in the pleural space usually denote this complication in the absence of an open drain. Although very small fistulas may heal by systemic antibiotics and tube thoracostomy alone, most require open drainage. Some demand an open surgical procedure to close the defect or to resect devitalized tissue.

Bronchopleural fistula is a dreaded complication of pneumonectomy, indicating stump breakdown. The majority of these cases require repeat thoracotomy to close or patch the defect.

Tuberculous Empyema

In tuberculous empyema the fluid is usually thin and serous. Because relatively few organisms may be present in the fluid, a pleural biopsy may be required to make the diagnosis. These fluids usually need not be drained by chest tube. (Historically, thoracostomy in this setting was often complicated by bacterial empyema.) Nonetheless, a thick fluid, a bronchopleural fistula, and a mixed infection are indications for establishing continuous drainage.

SUGGESTED READINGS

1.   Bartlett JG, et al. Bacteriology and treatment of primary lung abscess. Am. Rev. Respir. Dis. 1974;109:510-18.

2.   Bartlett JG, Feingold SM. Anaerobic infections of the lung and pleural space. Am. Rev. Respir. Dis. 1974;110:56-77.

3.   Berger HW, Majia E. Tuberculous pleurisy. Chest 1973;63:88-92.

4.   Friedman PJ, Hellekant CA. Radiologic recognition of bronchopleural fistula. Radiology 1977;124:289-95.

5.   Kirby BD, et al. Legionnaires' Disease: report of sixty-five nosocomially acquired cases and a review of the literature. Medicine 1980;59:188-205.

6.   LaForce FM. Hospital acquired gram-negative rod pneumonias: an overview. Am. J. Med. 1981;70:664-69.

7.   MacFarlane JT, et al. Hospital study of adult community acquired pneumonia. Lancet 1982;2:255-58.

8. Murray PR, Washington JA. Microscopic and bacteriologic analysis of expectorated sputum. Mayo Clin. Proc. 1975;50:339-44.

9. Pennington JE. Respiratory Infections. New York: Raven, 1983.

10. Reyes MP. The aerobic gram-negative bacillary pneumonias. Med. Clin. North Am. 1980;64:363-83.

11. Schachter EN. Suppurative lung disease: old problems revisited. Clin. Chest Med. 1981;2:41-49.

12. Tuazon CU. Gram positive pneumonias. Med. Clin. North Am. 1980;64:343-61.

13. Verghese A, Berk SL. Bacterial pneumonia in the elderly. Medicine 1983;62:271-85.

14. Yu VL, et al. Legionnaires' disease: new clinical perspective from a prospective pneumonia study. Am. J. Med. 1982;73:357-61.

Chapter 32

Pneumonitis in the Immunosuppressed Host

Few problems present a greater diagnostic challenge than acute pulmonary infiltration in the immunocompromised host (CH). Patients in this category have primary, iatrogenic deficits of T-lymphocyte (cell-mediated), B-cell (antibody), or granulocyte (phagocytic) function. Knowledge of the type of deficit can help to narrow the differential diagnosis. For example, T-cell disorders predispose to viruses and fungi and B-cell disorders to bacterial pathogens. Definitive treatment, however, requires a specific diagnosis. Because such patients often have impaired function of multiple organ systems or are under treatment with toxic agents, possible etiologies span a wide range of noninfectious and infectious causes. Multiple causes frequently coexist.

NONINFECTIOUS INFILTRATES

The major categories of noninfectious infiltrates in the CH include malignant involvement, lung edema, hemorrhage, drug reaction, and transfusion reaction.

Malignancy

Solid tumors frequently metastasize to the lung but uncommonly cause diagnostic confusion because of their circumscribed nature. On the other hand, lymphomas often behave in a nondescript fashion, with the range of involvement varying from circumscribed nodules and lymphadenopathy to diffuse infiltration and pleural effusion. In the untreated patient with leukemia, noninfectious pulmonary infiltrates usually derive from leukemic infiltration or parenchymal hemorrhage. Acute leukemic infiltrates are most common in the nonlymphocytic variants. Conversely, in the chronic group, malignant infiltration is most commonly seen in chronic lymphocytic leukemia.

Hemorrhage

Any disease or treatment that severely depresses platelet function can be associated with parenchymal hemorrhage. Leukemia, however is the most frequent predisposition to hemorrhagic infiltration. Unless strongly suspected, focal or diffuse parenchymal hemorrhage may escape clinical detection until biopsy, lung lavage, or autopsy confirm it. Hemoptysis occurs in fewer than half of all patients with parenchymal bleeding. Hemorrhage often mimics infection. Mild fever, impaired gas exchange, and constitutional complaints are frequent associations. An important clue to a hemorrhagic etiology is that platelet counts are almost always $< 20,000/mm^3$. Effective treatment centers on correction of the coagulopathy and supportive treatment.

Drug- and Radiation-Induced Lung Injury

The therapy used against neoplastic disease can induce parenchymal injury by cytotoxic and noncytotoxic mechanisms. Cytotoxic reactions produce bizarre atypia of the type 2 cells of the alveolar lining. Progression to disability and death may occur even after the offending agent is withdrawn. Currently, it is believed that injury is mediated, at least in part, by oxygen radicals. High inspired levels of oxygen can exacerbate the problem. Noncytotoxic reactions (typified by methotrexate) occur much less frequently and are associated with only a few types of drug. Noncytotoxic reactions are not associated with cellular atypia, are rarely fatal, and are usually self-limiting. Often, blood eosinophilia is present. From a clinician's standpoint the more common cytotoxic reactions can present a confusing picture.

The insidious onset of nonproductive cough, cyanosis, dyspnea, and fever 1-6 months after the onset of treatment is a typical presentation. The toxicity of some chemotherapeutic agents is clearly related to the total dose given. For example, cumulative doses of bleomycin exceeding 450 mg are attended by a high incidence of involvement. Bilateral infiltration, usually but not always symmetric, is the characteristic radiographic picture. The diagnosis is one of exclusion. A presumptive diagnosis can usually be made by transbronchoscopic biopsy and lavage, together with a typical clinical presentation. Supportive care, withdrawal of the offending agent, and corticosteroids are standard treatment for both types of problem.

Radiation pneumonitis is associated with histologic changes similar to those produced by cytotoxic chemotherapy, and the mechanism may be similar as well. The time course of onset parallels that of drug-induced disease. Interestingly, cytotoxic drugs (e.g., Cytoxan) appear to accelerate or intensify radiation effects when given before radiotherapy is begun. Tissue damage is generally confined to the irradiated field, so that even high doses of regional radiation may not produce symptoms, as the remaining lung is able to compensate. Sharp margins of infiltration are characteristic of radiation fibrosis but somewhat less so for acute pneumonitis. The schedule of dosing may be just as important as the total dose administered. Smaller, frequent doses are better tolerated than an identical cumulative dose given at a rapid rate. The treatment of radiation pneumonitis is largely supportive. Corticosteroids may be helpful, but no well-controlled prospective studies on this topic have been published to date.

Other Noninfectious Sources of Pulmonary Infiltration

A wide variety of ARDS-like reactions have been described in response to leukoagglutinins (following transfusion), during postchemotherapy tumor lysis, and idiosyncratically after receiving certain chemotherapeutic agents, e.g., cytosine arabinoside. Pulmonary infiltration in patients receiving chemotherapy or immunosuppresive agents can also result from a variety of factors indirectly related to the primary disease or its definitive treatment. Fluid overload is common in kidney transplant recipients, those receiving nephrotoxic drugs, and those with underlying cardiac disease. Pulmonary emboli and aspiration are frequent problems of all critically ill patients.

INFECTIOUS INFILTRATES

Although virtually any organism can cause pulmonary infiltration in the compromised host, the clinician can often integrate knowledge of the epidemiology, immune defect, and clinical and laboratory data to narrow the likely possibilities to a restricted number. A logical approach to diagnosis can then be formulated. As a first consideration, the underlying disease may give some clue to the nature of the pathogen, as granulocytopenia, T-lymphocyte dysfunction (lymphoma), B-cell dysfunction (myeloma, CLL), and splenectomy predispose to specific classes of organism.

For example, AIDS, a problem of helper T-lymphocytes, so predisposes to pneumocystis, mycobacterial, and cytomegalovirus infections that a presumptive diagnosis can often be made with confidence from the radiographic picture alone. Nonetheless, although somewhat helpful, this concept of "selective deficiency" is so often violated that the spectrum of possibilities remains widely open until biopsy confirmation.

Epidemiologic factors are also important to consider. Exposures to unusual organisms can occur through travel, interaction with infective carriers, or blood transfusion. The duration of hospitalization prior to the development of pneumonitis influences the microbiology. For example, pseudomonas, candida, and aspergillus infections are most likely to develop after many days in hospital, whereas consideration of community-acquired pneumonias wanes rapidly in importance after the first few days of confinement. Renal transplant recipients are usually prone to cytomegalovirus, herpes symplex, cryptococcous, aspergillus, and pneumocystis carini infections during the period of maximal T-cell suppression, 1-6 months after operation. Neutropenic patients, such as those undergoing chemotherapy for leukemia, are highly susceptible to Gram-negative bacteria and fungal infections (aspergillus, zygomycetes).

Concurrent infection of two or more organisms occurs commonly in patients with AIDS and recent renal or marrow transplantation. Cytomegalovirus, cryptococcus, and nocardia are frequently recovered in conjunction with other pathogens. (Cytomegalovirus and pneumocystis is a common association.) Superinfections are also frequent in immunosuppressed patients, particularly during sustained neutropenia, prolonged high-dose immunosuppressive therapy, and following thromboembolic events.

Certain clinical findings are especially noteworthy. Cryptococcosis, nocardia, mycobacteria, and varicella are the most common causes of concurrent pulmonary and CNS disease in patients with T-cell dysfunction. Legionella, strongyloides, and cryptosporidium are common offenders when diarrhea coexists with pulmonary infiltration. Skin lesions and infiltrates are a common association for pseudomonas, aspergillus, candida, and varicella-zoster infections. Hepatic and pulmonary disease tend to coexist during cytomegalovirus, nocardial, mycobacterial necrotizing bacterial (pseudemonas, staphylococcal) infections.

Diagnostic Workup

In these seriously ill patients a wide variety of infectious and noninfectious problems may be responsible for pulmonary infiltration. The pace of the disease may proceed very rapidly, so that the objective is to achieve a specific etiologic diagnosis expediently and safely. Unfortunately, these problems often defy rapid diagnosis, and a tissue biopsy is frequently needed to establish a diagnosis.

Ancillary Data

Both the characteristics of the chest x-ray at any single point in time and its rate of progression can provide helpful diagnostic clues. Localized infiltrates, either consolidated or nodular, are most consistent with bacterial or fungal infection, hemorrhage, or thromboembolic disease. Bilateral "interstitial" infiltrates, on the other hand, suggest volume-overload pneumocystis, mycobacterial, or viral processes. It is important to realize that a serious lung infection may be established even without pulmonary infiltrates. A fulminant evolution suggests a bacterial process or a non-infective etiology (fluid overload, embolism, ARDS). Conversely, a process requiring 1-2 weeks for full expression calls to mind mycobacterial parasitic or systemic fungal diseases. Another key finding is the severity of hypoxemia.

Life-threatening depressions of blood oxygen tension are typical for bacterial, viral, and pneumocystis infections but are uncommon with fungal and mycobacterial processes.

Examination of body fluids other than those from a pulmonary source can be useful, but even when positive allow for only a presumptive diagnosis of the chest infiltrate. For example, spinal fluid may demonstrate cryptococcus but does not prove that the roentgenographic infiltrates are related. Nonetheless, pleural and joint fluid should be tapped, examined, and cultured and a stool specimen sent for evaluation and parasite detection. Blood cultures are unquestionably important, whereas serologic testing rarely provides definitive information in an appropriate time frame.

Pulmonary Secretions and Tissue

Sputum is less frequently produced by the CH than by immunocompetent patients, especially when neutropenia is present. Nonetheless, when sputum can be obtained, its careful examination may reveal the responsible pathogen. Apart from the routine Gram stain, a direct fluorescent antibody test for legionella, a phase contrast or cytologic preparation for blastomycosis, an acid-fast stain for mycobacteria and nocardia, and a silver stain for pneumocystis and fungal elements are highly worthwhile. Concentrated specimens may reveal strongyloides. Patients with AIDS harbor such a profusion of pneumocystis organisms that expectorated specimens often reveal them. Unfortunately, cultures of many pathogens of interest require days to weeks for confirmation.

In attempting to deal effectively with a life-threatening pulmonary process in a compromised host there are, perhaps, two primary questions. First, given that a process appears to be infectious and that the diagnosis cannot be made easily, does a precise diagnosis need to be established? (Is empiric therapy sufficient?) Second, if a precise diagnosis is required, what is the most efficacious technique in a fragile, critically ill patient? These questions are not straightforward and remain the subject of intense controversy. In general, the approach should vary with the severity of illness, the pace of advancement, the coagulation and ventilation status, the strength of ancillary information, and the experience of available personnel with specific invasive procedures. If a diffuse pattern on CXR cannot be confidently distinguished from pulmonary edema, a brief trial of diuresis may be prudent before proceeding to invasive measures aimed at documenting infection. "Diuresis before biopsy" is a good rule of thumb. Sputum examination, when possible, is an obvious first step. Transtracheal aspiration and transthoracic needle biopsy are dangerous, low-yield procedures in this setting and should be withheld.

Biopsy

If a specific diagnosis is not in hand after review of clinical data and laboratory results, the next step should be guided by the strength of the clinical suspicion and the urgency of making the correct diagnosis. In most instances bronchoscopy should be employed as the first invasive procedure. Although coagulopathy and the need for mechanical ventilation are strong relative contraindications to forceps biopsy, lavage and gentle brushings can be safely obtained when care is taken to administer platelets and/or missing clotting components beforehand. Bronchoscopic yield varies greatly with the disease process and with the method of conducting this procedure. For example, when all specimen-gathering techniques (biopsy, brushings, and lavage) are used, a specific diagnosis can be established in about 50% of cases. In special instances, such as AIDS, the yield is considerably higher.

The decision to undertake an open lung biopsy is often delayed because of the perceived morbidity and expense of the procedure when compared to empiric multidrug treatment. In fact, open biopsy when conducted early in the course of the illness is well tolerated, safe, and helfpul. Open biopsy is a procedure that can be completed within 20-40 minutes. It is the only truly safe method of establishing effective hemostasis in patients at high risk for bleeding and often provides sufficient tissue to make a histologic diagnosis. Its expense should be considered alongside the expense of empiric multi-antibiotic therapy, which can easily mount to a similar value. The antibiotics commonly used (trimethoprim sulfa, aminoglycosides, amphotericin) are not without associated toxicity for kidneys and bone marrow. Whatever the value of open lung biopsy may be when undertaken early in the course of disease, it is clearly less valuable after broad spectrum antibiotics have been given over a prolonged period. In such instances it is unusual for open biopsy to add sufficient new information to warrant its attendant drawbacks.

Antibiotic management can be streamlined when a specific diagnosis has been made. However, the clinician must remain alert for the development of superinfection. When no specific diagnosis has been made and the clinician is forced to choose a regimen, it should be remembered that legionella and pneumocystis are among the most lethal and common pathogens. In addition to a third-generation cephalosporin and an aminoglycoside, erythromycin and trimethoprim sulfa are usually chosen. In centers where fungi have proven a major problem, amphotericin is often begun very early in the course. The recent introduction of ultrabroad spectrum antibiotics (such as imipenim) may help to greatly simplify initial coverage.

SUGGESTED READINGS

1.   Blank N, Castellino RA, Shah V.   Radiologic aspects of pulmonary infection in patients with altered immunity. Radiol. Clin. North Am. 1973;11:175-90.

2.   Fanta CH, Pennington JE. Fever and new lung infiltrates in the immunocompromised host. Clin. Chest Med. 1981;2:19-39.

3.   Gross NJ. Pulmonary effects of radiation therapy. Ann. Int. Med. 1977;86:81-92.

4.   McCabe RE, Brooks RG.   Open lung biopsy in patients with acute leukemia. Am. J. Med. 1985;78:609-16.

5.   Murray JF, et al.   Pulmonary complications of the acquired immunodeficiency syndrome. N. Engl. J. Med. 1984;310:1682-88.

6.   Rosenow EC, Wilson WR, Cockerill FR.   Pulmonary disease in the immunocompromised host. Mayo Clin. Proc. 1985;60:473-87, 610-31.

7.   Stover DE, et al.   Bronchoalveolar lavage in the diagnosis of diffuse pulmonary infiltrates in the immunosuppressed host.   Ann. Int. Med. 1984;101:1-7.

8.   Weiss RB, Muggia FM.   Cytotoxic drug-induced pulmonary disease. Update 1980. Am. J. Med. 1980;68:259-66.

9.   Williams D, et al. The role of fiberoptic bronchoscopy in the evaluation of immunocompromised hosts with diffuse pulmonary infiltrates.   Am. Rev. Respir. Dis. 1985;131:880-85.

10.   Williams DM, Krick JA, Remington JS.   Pulmonary infection in the compromised host. Am. Rev. Respir. Dis. 1976;114:359-94, 593-627.

Chapter 33

Restrictive Lung Disease

RESTRICTIVE DISEASES OF THE LUNG PARENCHYMA

General Characteristics of Restrictive Disease

Disorders of the chest wall and muscular pump have been considered in Chapter 26. This chapter addresses the broad spectrum of diseases that limit chest expansion by reducing the effective compliance of the lung itself. Any problem that reduces the number of aerated alveoli (pneumonectomy, atelectasis, alveolar flooding or filling) or that impairs the distensibility of aerated units (granulomatous or fibrous interstitial processes) increases the energy cost of lung expansion and acts to limit lung volume. Because resting lung volume during passive exhalation is determined by the joint tendencies of the chest wall to spring outward and the lung parenchyma to retract, pulmonary function testing in parenchymal disease reveals more or less symmetrical reductions in RV, FRC, and TLC. The normal breathing pattern is altered in favor of a more energy-efficient pattern, with minute ventilation accomplished by a combination of higher frequency and lower tidal volume.

Idiopathic Pulmonary Fibrosis	Collagen Vascular	Drug/Radiation
Usual Interstitial Fibrosis	Systemic Lupus	Nitrofurantoin
Desquamative Interstitial Fib.	Rheumatoid	Cytotoxic Agents
Lymphocytic Interstitial Fib.	Scleroderma	Gold
Bronchiolitis Obliterans	Derm/Polymyositis	Radio Rx
	Mixed Connective	

Granulomatous	Miscellaneous
Sarcoidosis	Carcinomatosis
Hypersensitivity	Eosinophilic Granuloma
Infections	Neurofibromatosis
	Tuberous Sclerosis

$D_L CO$ is invariably reduced and usually remains so when referenced to aerated lung volume (D_L/V_A). Arterial blood gases generally reveal hypoxemia that worsens during exercise. Pulmonary hypertension is a frequent concomitant. Many patients with restrictive lung disease maintain a mild respiratory alkalosis $(PaCO_2 < 40$ mmHg$)$, presumably driven by enhanced sensory input from pulmonary receptors.

Whatever the etiology, patients with parenchymal restriction commonly present with symptoms of limited exercise tolerance and dyspnea. The physical examination is noteworthy for basilar late-inspiratory crepitations, tachypnea, and cyanosis in most patients, but these findings are not invariably present. Other physical findings characteristic of the underlying etiology may give important clues.

Selected Diseases

Sarcoidosis

Although its etiology remains unknown, sarcoidosis is believed to represent an unusual reaction to an inhaled irritant or allergen. With or without x-ray evidence, the lungs and the lymphatic system draining the lungs are involved in virtually all documented cases, often representing the sole manifestation of the disease. Radiographically sarcoidosis can be classified in 3 categories or "stages": 1) hilar adenopathy without x-ray evidence of parenchymal involvement, 2) combined hilar adenopathy and infiltrative disease, and 3) pulmonary infiltrates without hilar disease. It should be emphasized that the x-ray manifestations are protean, ranging from diffuse bilateral infiltrates to focal, nodular cavitating disease. Bilateral adenopathy is the rule, but unilateral disease may occur in 5-10% of cases. Although there is a general tendency for patients in categories 2 and 3 to have evolved through Stage 1, it is not clear that all patients do so. Furthermore, the great majority of affected persons do not progress beyond Stage 1, which characteristically is associated with few symptoms and may therefore often escape detection. A significant majority of patients, perhaps 25-50%, become overtly symptomatic with constitutional complaints of unexplained fever, diaphoresis, weight loss, hypercalcemia, exercise limitation, erythema nodosum, and eye, joint, or (rarely) vital organ involvement. Although usually a self-limited disease, an unfortunate minority of patients progress inexorably to severe end-organ damage or death. Bilateral hilar adenopathy, particularly when accompanied by paratracheal nodal involvement and clear separation of "potato-like" hilar nodes from more proximal mediastinal structures, is highly characteristic. With such a picture, asymptomatic cases, or those accompanied by uveoparotid symptomatology or erythema nodosum, can generally be observed closely or treated presumptively, without tissue confirmation. However, any departure from a classical presentation or course (e.g., anemia) warrants a more invasive approach. In the absence of overt disease in accessible tissues (nodes, skin), bronchoscopy with transbronchial biopsy and lavage is highly productive; noncaseating granulomata can be demonstrated by transbronchial biopsy in approximately 2/3 of cases without, and 5/6 of those with, x-ray involvement of the lung. Lavage demonstrates a profusion of helper T-lymphocytes in active cases and can be used as corroborating data. Active sarcoid tissue is gallium avid and generates angiotensin-converting enzyme (ACE) in large quantities. These tests provide helpful indications of disease activity and response to therapy but must not be viewed in themselves as definitive diagnostic data.

Sarcoidosis generally runs a self-limited course over a few months to years. Granulomatous inflammation tends to respond well to corticosteroid treatment in modest doses, which can often be tapered rapidly to very small maintenance doses. Therefore, I believe that unless strong contraindications exist, a therapeutic trial of corticosteroids should be initiated in the great majority of patients with symptomatic disease, tapering to the lowest dosage that maintains remission over a period of several months.

Idiopathic Pulmonary Fibrosis (IPF)

Another group of parenchymal restrictive diseases of unknown origin have been classified together on the basis of predominance in the lung and clinical presentation. These disorders have been termed cryptogenic fibrosing alveolitis, idiopathic interstitial pneumonitis, and diffuse interstitial fibrosis. Although there are some clear histologic differences, these disorders share a common clinical presentation, diagnostic approach, and therapeutic strategy and therefore are profitably considered together. Useful pathologic distinctions may be made on the basis of the nature of the cellular infiltrate as well as the relative exuberance of cellular and fibrotic response. The two most common variants are usual interstitial pneumonitis (UIP), characterized histologically by mononuclear and polymorphonuclear infiltrates and variable degrees of fibrosis, and desquamative interstitial pneumonitis (DIP), whose pathology is characterized by a more impressive mononuclear cellular infiltrate, without major fibrosis in the interstitial regions, and cellular proliferation in the alveolar space. DIP tends to be more steroid responsive than UIP and may in some patients simply represent an unusually exuberant first phase of the UIP process. Other pathologic variants of interstitial fibrosis (the lymphocytic and giant cell interstitial pneumonias) are much less common.

All categories of IPF tend to share certain characteristic features. They tend to develop in late middle age and begin insidiously with dyspnea on exertion, easy fatigability, and nonproductive cough. Cyanosis may be evident from the outset. Physical examination is also notable for late inspiratory basilar crepitations and digital clubbing. Although the chest roentgenogram may be unremarkable except for reduced lung volumes, diffuse fibrosis with basilar predominance is more common. (This pattern is also observed in chronic aspiration pneumonia - an important differential diagnosis with a similar clinical presentation but a wholly different therapeutic approach.) Late in the disease, the classical appearance of honeycomb lung may be evident. Apart from the symmetrical reduction of lung volumes common to all restrictive diseases, rates of airflow corrected for lung volume tend to be high, as enhanced elasticity increases the tractive forces on the airway and boosts the alveolar pressure driving airflow.

The pace of this disease is highly variable. Most patients follow a slowly inexorable course to death over a period of 3-5 years. Yet there is extreme variation, ranging from an accelerated 6-month course (the Hamman-Rich syndrome) to a disease process that "burns out" over a protracted period. The symptomatic onset of overt cor pulmonale usually signals the approach of the terminal phase. Diagnosis rests on biopsy evidence, together with a compatible clinical course.

Transbronchoscopic biopsy and lavage usually enable a presumptive diagnosis but seldom yield sufficient tissue to settle the issue when the clinical presentation is confusing. Open biopsy is a better choice in those instances where atypical clinical features suggest an alternative diagnosis, such as vasculitis, or where there are relative contraindications to immunosuppressive therapy. A relatively cellular biopsy encourages a trial of corticosteroids, the treatment of first choice. Cyclophosphamide or azathioprine may be added or substituted if the response is suboptimal. Immunosuppression should be withdrawn if no response is evident. Oxygen therapy may help symptomatically and may be effective in reducing the severity and rate of progression of pulmonary hypertension.

Collagen Vascular Diseases

Rheumatoid arthritis is associated with a profusion of lung disorders, including pleural effusions, pleural fibrosis, sterile empyema, necrobiotic nodules, pulmonary hypertension, and diffusely fibrotic lung disease. Interestingly, males appear to be more susceptible to rheumatoid lung disease, even though the disease itself is most common in females.

The interstitial pneumonitis of rheumatoid arthritis has two primary variants. The first is virtually indistinguishable from idiopathic pulmonary fibrosis and should be approached in a similar fashion. It appears, however, to be even less responsive to immunosuppressive drug therapy. The second has a prominent component of associated small airway disease that can progress to bronchiolitis obliterans, a disorder associated with profound hypoxemia, dyspnea, and resistance to drug treatment. A wholly obstructive, restrictive, or mixed functional abnormality may be evident.

Granulomatous Vasculitis (Wegener's and its variants) - Wegener's is the most common among a group of restrictive disorders whose shared pathologic feature is granulomatous vasculitis. Full-blown Wegener's is a generalized systemic disease that typically involves the upper respiratory tract, the lungs, and the kidneys, whereas overt damage from its more benign variant tends to be limited to the lung. Patients come to clinical attention for varied reasons. When referable to the respiratory tract, symptoms tend to be those related to pain or discharge of abnormal nasal or pulmonary secretions: e.g., sinus drainage, cough, hemoptysis, otitis, etc. Exercise-related dyspnea or generalized breathlessness are much less characteristic of Wegener's than of IPF. Indeed, mortality is much more commonly related to renal than to pulmonary failure.

The chest x-ray is also highly variable. Diffuse symmetrical infiltration is uncommon. Rather, localized infiltrates and nodules are more characteristic. Infiltrates tend to be fleeting, with some regions improving while others simultaneously worsen. The lymph nodes of the hilum and mediastinum are not involved. Upon pulmonary function evaluation, the usual picture is restrictive; however, an obstructive pattern may be seen when central airways are compressed. Definitive diagnosis requires a substantial biopsy from involved tissue. Bronchoscopic findings are seldom more than suggestive. Only open biopsy can provide the vascular tissue required to make the diagnosis of an angiocentric disorder. Whereas corticosteroids may be helpful as initial therapy in some cases of Wegener's, cyclophosphamide is clearly the drug of choice. It appears that the majority of cases can be controlled with this drug, and long-term survival is the rule for this once devastating and fulminant disease.

Other forms of granulomatous vasculitis noted for their pulmonary component include the Churg-Strauss (CS) syndrome (allergic granulomatosis), lymphomatoid granulomatosis, and bronchocentric granulomatosis. The CS syndrome is typified by a strong allergic background history, dense eosinophilic infiltration, and peripheral eosinophilia. Cutaneous and joint symptoms are more prominent and renal disorders are less prominent than with Wegener's. The x-ray appearance is comparable. Unlike Wegener's, corticosteroids, not cyclophosphamide, are the treatment of choice. Bronchocentric granulomatosis (BG) is often considered to be in the Wegener's group but may in fact represent a different process altogether. Like those with the CS syndrome, patients with BG have a strong allergic prehistory and chest x-rays that mimic Wegener's. Histologically the infiltrate is bronchocentric, not angiocentric, in nature, however, and the disease responds better to corticosteroids than to cyclophosphamide. Allergic aspergillosis may be an inciting factor in many instances. Finally, lymphomatoid granulomatosis (LG) appears to be a Wegener's variant that primarily affects the lung and less commonly the skin and nervous system. Atypical lymphocytes are the hallmark of its angiocentric infiltrate, and degeneration to lymphoma is common. This disease is cyclophosphamide responsive. LG should be distinguished therapeutically and prognostically from lymphocytic angitis and granulomatosis, a benign disease that generally remains confined to the lung. The mature lymphocytes that compose its infiltrate respond well to treatment with chlorambucil.

Systemic Lupus Erythematosus, Scleroderma, Polymyositis, and Mixed Connective Tissue Disease - Systemic lupus erythematosus (SLE) presents frequently and in a varied fashion within the lung. Apart from infections, pleuritis, and pleural effusion, the lung may be primarily affected by lupus pneumonitis, diffuse interstitial disease, and diaphragmatic dysfunction with attendant lower lobe collapse or generalized volume loss. Each problem presents a restrictive picture. Acute lupus pneumonitis is an acute process that presents with fever, cough, tachypnea, and hypoxemia. The chest x-ray is notable for irregular areas of increased density. The process may resolve spontaneously or under steroid, azathioprine, or cyclophosphamide therapy. Radiographic infiltrates may persist once symptoms abate, blending into the picture of chronic interstitial pneumonitis. Diffuse bilateral interstitial disease is considerably less common than pleural disease, atelectasis, or acute pneumonitis. Pulmonary function tests reveal impaired $D_L CO$ and reduced lung volumes. Respiratory muscle strength is impaired in many patients with SLE, believed secondary to a diffuse myopathy. Basilar atelectasis, generalized loss of lung volume ("shrinking lungs"), and marked orthopnea tend to characterize this process.

Progressive systemic sclerosis (PSS) is not generally thought of as a lung disorder because it rarely presents dramatically as such, but most patients eventually develop pathologic evidence of pulmonary involvement. As in SLE, $D_L CO$ and lung volume testing reveal dysfunction in nearly all cases of advanced disease, even when there is little clinical or roentgenographic evidence of impairment. Both vascular lesions and interstitial fibrosis may appear, generally quite independently of one another. Recurrent aspiration pneumonia may contribute to the basilar fibrosis. Exertional dyspnea is a common complaint, due both to restrictive disease and pulmonary hypertension. Open lung biopsy is seldom needed to make a presumptive diagnosis, as other problems characteristic of PSS are usually manifest before the need for a pulmonary diagnosis arises. Furthermore, treatment of the lung disease of PSS is supportive for pulmonary hypertension (oxygen) and prophylactic against aspiration (positioning, antibiotics). Corticosteroids and cytotoxic agents have not been shown to be beneficial in this illness.

Polymyositis and dermatomyositis are much less commonly associated with lung pathology than are SLE or PSS, but the manifestations are similar. Muscular weakness predisposes to hypoventilation, atelectasis, and aspiration pneumonia. On chest x-ray, lower lobe infiltrates tend to predominate. Interstitial pneumonitis, similar in character to PSS, also occurs. Unlike PSS, however, the lung disorder often precedes the onset of disease elsewhere. The lung disorders of polymyositis and dermatomyositis, again unlike PSS, often respond to corticosteroids.

Mixed connective tissue disease can manifest in a fashion similar to SLE, PSS, or polymyositis, and the spectrum lung pathology is similar. The course of the lung disease and the response to corticosteroids tend to follow the course of the disease it most resembles.

SUGGESTED READINGS

1. Crystal RG, et al. Interstitial lung disease of unknown cause: disorders characterized by chronic inflammation of the lower respiratory tract. N. Engl. J. Med. 1984;310:154-66, 235-44.

2. Fauci AS, et al. Wegener's granulomatosis: prospective clinical and therapeutic experience with 85 patients for 21 years. Ann. Int. Med. 1983;98:76-85.

3. Fulmer JD, Kaltreider HB. The pulmonary vasculitides. Chest 1982;82:615-24.

4. Gross NJ. Pulmonary effects of radiation therapy. Ann. Int. Med. 1977;86:81-92.

5. Hunninghake GW, Fauci AS. Pulmonary involvement in the collagen vascular diseases. Am. Rev. Respir. Dis. 1979;119:471-503.

6. Rudd RM, Haslam PL, Turner-Warwick M. Cryptogenic fibrosing alveolitis: relationships of pulmonary physiology and bronchoalveolar lavage to response to treatment and prognosis. Am. Rev. Respir. Dis. 1981;124:1-8.

7. Thrasher DR, Briggs DD Jr. Pulmonary sarcoidosis. Clin. Chest Med. 1982;3:537-63.

Chapter 34

Sleep Apnea

CLASSIFICATION

Men and postmenopausal women are the groups at greatest risk for sleep apnea. Despite the prevalence of obesity in affected persons, sleep apnea can affect persons of any body habitus. As recognition of the problem developed, episodes of airflow cessation during sleep were classified according to mechanism: Obstructive. The retropharyngeal muscles relax to occlude the upper airway despite continued ventilatory efforts. Central. Nerve traffic to the respiratory musculature ceases so that no respiratory efforts occur. Complex (mixed). Apneic periods are characterized by features of both.

PATHOPHYSIOLOGY

Although the genesis of sleep apnea remains poorly understood, both central and obstructive variants are considered to be of CNS origin. Obstructive apnea occurs when the dilatory muscles of the upper airway fail to resist the negative pressure generated during breathing efforts. Many structural disorders of the neck and oropharynx predispose to obstructive sleep apnea, including obesity, myxedema, acromegaly, goiter, micrognathia, and adenotonsillar hypertrophy. Apart from anatomic narrowing of the airway, the pharynx of these persons appears to be unusually collapsible during sleep, unable to resist the closing pressure developed within the airway during inspiration. Therefore, anything that accentuates the negative pressure within the thorax (nasal obstruction, vigorous respiratory efforts) is likely to cause problems in the predisposed.

During an obstructive episode, the patient makes increasingly vigorous attempts to ventilate, a sequence that culminates in a powerful effort and a loud snort as obstruction is transiently relieved. The effort rouses the patient to near consciousness, and normal breathing resumes only to be interrupted moments later in a similar fashion. Cyclical hypoxemia, mild acidosis, and stress raise pulmonary vascular resistance and provoke arrhythmias. Although it is unproven whether sleep apnea alone is sufficient to cause cor pulmonale, the clinical association is undeniable. In patients without the full-blown Pickwickian syndrome, waking ventilatory drives to hypoxemia and CO_2 appear to be nearly normal. During sleep, however, tolerance to hypoxemia and CO_2 is often extraordinary.

CLINICAL SYNDROMES

Many normal individuals experience brief episodes of apnea lasting 10-15 seconds at the onset of sleep or during REM. These are not disruptive to the cycle of sleep stages. Based upon data obtained in healthy adults, any number of 10-second apneic episodes that exceed 30 during a 7-hour sleep study period is statistically abnormal, provided that apnea occurs both during REM and non-REM phases. However, the patient with such an abnormality may or may not report symptoms. Symptomatic patients average hundreds of episodes nightly, many of very long duration.

The majority of patients with serious disorders are obese middle-aged men. (An interesting hypothesis is that obesity may be as much the result of the sedentary behavior that somnolence induces as the causal factor.) Thus, the earliest recognized example of sleep apnea - the Pickwickian syndrome of obesity, hypersomnolence, polycythemia, hypercapnia, and cor pulmonale - is perhaps the most fully developed example in a wide spectrum.

Memory loss, morning headaches, and sexual impotence may be the patient's major complaints. Intellectual impairment and personality changes are often noted by the family - a symptom complex suggestive of depression. Typical patients with sleep apnea usually present with crippling daytime somnolence, a manifestation of the fragmented nocturnal sleep pattern. Conversely, some complain primarily of nocturnal insomnia and only secondarily of daytime somnolence. The fraction of sleep time spent in stages 3 and 4, the deep non-REM phases, is always markedly reduced, whereas the fraction of REM sleep may be nearly normal. Visual hallucinations vivid enough to incite action often occur as the urge to sleep descends (hypnagogic hallucinations). Polycythemia and signs of pulmonary or systemic hypertension may be evident on physical examination. During sleep, the patient invariably exhibits loud snoring and agitated motor activity. Somnambulism, falling out of bed, or enuresis are frequently reported.

DIAGNOSIS

Suspicion is raised by a history of excessive daytime somnolence, in conjunction with reports from family members of loud snoring and agitated sleeping. Many patients who snore loudly do not obstruct the airway but produce noise at the level of the nasopharynx. Nonetheless, snoring is a good screening symptom, because very few patients with obstructive apnea do not snore loudly. In patients without somnolence, the disorder may go undiscovered for years, presenting subtly as unexplained pulmonary hypertension, deterioration of mental function, or insomnia.

Although the condition is often obvious by casual inspection of the sleepy patient, the diagnosis can only be confirmed by observing monitored sleep. To exclude obstructive sleep apnea, a study must last at least 6 hours and include at least two periods of fully developed REM. A minimum laboratory setup includes an indicator of airflow (nasal thermistor, CO_2 analyzer) and a measure of ventilatory effort (esophageal balloon, surface magnetometry, impedance plethysmography, electromyography of the respiratory musculature). Continuous noninvasive electrocardiographic and oxygen saturation monitoring are highly desirable. Serious arrhythmias and sudden death are common in patients with the full-blown disease. Electroencephalography and electro-oculography are useful to ensure that sleep has occurred, to apportion sleep stages, and to compare periods of apnea with those of eye movement. However, they are not essential, except for patients who have an atypical presentation of apnea. Most patients with hypersomnolence have no trouble sleeping, despite the discomfort of monitoring paraphernalia. Although more than 30 apneic periods of greater than 10 seconds duration provide a guideline for a positive study, no sharp criteria for the diagnosis exist. Many elderly persons would qualify for the diagnosis by this standard but are asymptomatic. Usually there is no doubt, because the studies of symptomatic patients are floridly positive.

DIAGNOSTIC WORKUP

History (patient and sleeping partner)
Sitting and supine arterial blood gases
CBC
Pulmonary function tests, including tests for structural upper airway obstruction
Ear, nose, and throat examination
Sleep study

MANAGEMENT

Therapy for the sleep-apnea syndromes depends upon the nature and intensity of symptoms and the mechanism of apnea. As experience has been gained, treatment options have expanded greatly in recent years. This disease can now be successfully approached by a variety of mechanical and surgical means.

Correctable anatomical aberrations that predispose to upper airway obstruction should be treated. Obese patients should be admonished to lose weight. However, this strategy meets with limited success; few lose weight, and weight losers sometimes retain their symptoms.

Persons with nasal obstruction may respond to an approach as simple as nasal decongestion. Because alcohol ingestion is documented to accentuate problems, alcoholic beverages must be prohibited. Stimulators of ventilatory drive (progesterone 20 mg t.i.d. or acetazolamide 125-250 mg HS) appear to be of little benefit but are worth a brief trial, especially in patients with a major component of central apnea. Nonsedating tricyclic antidepressants, such as protriptylene, are an effective adjunct for a minority of patients. In most patients nocturnal oxygen therapy will improve symptoms related to desaturation and occasionally those of hypersomnolence as well. (Oxygen supplementation can prolong the periods of apnea in some patients, but the clinical implications of this have not been clearly defined.) Changing the sleep posture to lateral or prone does not appear to stop obstructive episodes.

In recent years, two innovations have made a major impact: nasal CPAP and surgical modification of the oropharynx. Nasal CPAP splints open the collapsible upper airway with gentle pressure, maintaining patency. It appears that nasal CPAP is effective for the majority of patients in whom it is conscientiously tried and is certainly worth considering before more aggressive measures are attempted. Some authorities suggest a nasal CPAP trial before any other approach. From anecdotal reports, the recently introduced indwelling transtracheal oxygen catheter provides another exciting but as yet untested approach. When effective, it may act both by supplementing oxygen and by an airway splinting mechanism. Surgical reconstruction procedures (uvulopharyngopalatoplasty) involve submucosal resection of redundant tissue from the pharyngeal inlet and can be remarkably effective in some, but by no means all, patients. Finally, bypassing the upper airway with tracheostomy generally improves somnolence and hypoxemia dramatically-within a day or two in most patients. Rare patients with refractory disease may require nocturnal positive-pressure ventilation.

SUGGESTED READINGS

1.   Block AJ, et al.   Factors influencing upper airway closure.   Chest 1984;86:114-22.

2.   Cherniack NS.   Respiratory dysrhythmias during sleep.   N. Engl. J. Med. 1981;305:325-30.

3.   Strohl KP, Cherniack NS, Gothe B.   Physiologic basis of therapy for sleep apnea.   State of Art.   Am. Rev. Respir. Dis.   1986;134:791-802.

4.   Sullivan CE, Issa FG.   Obstructive sleep apnea.   Clin. Chest Med. 1985;6:633-50.

Chapter 35

Tuberculosis and Fungal Diseases of the Lung

TUBERCULOSIS

PATHOGENESIS

Innoculation with Mycobacterium tuberculosis occurs when an infected microdroplet settles deep within the lung, often in a lower lobe. Although the local reaction is usually (95%) completely asymptomatic, widespread lymphohematogenous dissemination occurs, seeding favorable organ sites with viable organisms. As these organisms multiply, they induce the delayed hypersensitivity that arrests the process and provides a slowly waning resistance to exogenous reinfection.

In a small number of persons (especially the very young or immunosuppressed), symptomatic bronchopneumonia develops directly following inoculation ("primary infection"). This bronchopneumonia usually heals spontaneously, but a weak immune response may allow progression to massive tissue necrosis or simultaneous active infection of multiple extrapulmonary organs (miliary spread).

The vast majority of persons with asymptomatic reactions form granulomas around minute foci that remain stable throughout life, despite their load of viable organisms. However, in approximately one patient in 20, host defenses are eventually overcome. This breakdown causes "secondary" disease in pulmonary or extrapulmonary sites, by far the most common form of active tuberculosis (TB) in the United States. (It should be noted that the incidence of re-activation of an original focus declines progressively with time after innoculation, but susceptibility to new infection increases again after a period of years.) Approximately 30% of patients with ongoing disease are not sufficiently symptomatic to seek medical attention, and TB is discovered incidentally during screening programs, etc. In the preantibiotic era, approximately 1/2 of those with secondary infection died from the illness, 1/4 eventually had their disease arrested (with recurrences), and 1/4 experienced a chronically active process.

DIAGNOSIS

Skin Testing

Skin test hypersensitivity develops 2-6 weeks after exposure and persists throughout life, waning somewhat in advanced age. In infected persons, intradermal inoculation of purified protein tuberculin antigens (PPD) causes noticeable induration within 48-72 hours. However, sensitization to innocuous "atypical" mycobacteria is frequent in certain regions of the country, especially the South and Southeast. Hypersensitivity to these atypical organisms causes cross-reactions with the standard "intermediate" (5 TU) strength of PPD, usually of 5 mm or less. The frequency and size of these nonspecific reactions are greater with 250 TU (second-strength) PPD.

Hence, it is necessary for practical purposes to define a "positive" reaction as induration exceeding 10 mm in greatest diameter following a standard 5 TU dose. On sequential testing, "conversion" from negative to positive is said to occur if induration increases by 6 mm or more to a size of 10 mm or greater. Nonetheless, reactions less than 10 mm may be evidence of active tuberculosis in some debilitated or immunosuppressed patients or may indicate long-quiescent infection in older, healthy persons. Doubtful reactions (5-9 mm) should not be considered negative in patients who appear to have active disease, who are contacts of active cases, or who have always lived in geographic areas with low incidence of atypicals.

In certain older patients mere administration of PPD is sufficient to re-awaken the dormant delayed response, so that rechallenge with PPD may elicit a greater reaction one week to one month later. The magnitude of this "booster" effect is a direct function of advancing age. The phenomenon is rare if the second dose is given sooner than one week or later than several months after the first test. Amplified reactions occurring outside that time range are more likely to reflect an error of initial administration (if earlier) or a new infection (if later).

Falsely negative tests may occur in patients with generalized anergy due to malnutrition, viral disease, overwhelming illness, or immune compromise. "False negatives" due to selective anergy to tuberculin protein rarely occur. Although skin tests can be done with the tine or Heaf methods, the dose administered is less certain than with intradermal needle injection, and doubtful or positive results should be verified with the Mantoux technique.

Smears and Cultures

Tuberculosis should be strongly suspected if a sputum smear shows numerous acid-fast organisms of typical appearance (beaded outline, asymmetrical staining, tendency to occur in pairs). Unfortunately, organisms are often difficult to demonstrate, and false positives occur frequently, especially with fluorochrome stains.

Because sputum may be positive intermittently, at least three specimens should be obtained (and concentrated) before assuming smear negativity. If the patient cannot produce sputum spontaneously, a trial of cough induction by ultrasonic nebulization of saline should be tried. When suspicion remains strong, and sputum cannot be obtained, the fiberoptic bronchoscope can be used to sample tissue from the area involved radiographically. Acid-fast contaminants occur frequently in gastric aspirates, and the number of organisms recovered is very small. Hence, most laboratories refuse to do acid-fast smears on such material.

Therapy should be started in very ill patients with suspected tuberculosis, even as efforts to secure specimens proceed. (Chemotherapy will not sterilize cultures for several days to weeks after it is initiated.) Extrapulmonary disease (which has remained stable in its incidence as pulmonary tuberculosis has declined) must be diagnosed by examination of tissues or fluids obtained from the involved organs.

Smears alone miss 60% of active cases of TB. Culture of multiple colonies of niacin-positive organisms is the only definitive method to establish the diagnosis on conventional media. Although standard cultures require 2-6 weeks to grow on standard media, newer liquid medium culture techniques may allow identification in 10 days or less. Fewer than 5 colonies on solid media usually indicate either contamination of the specimen in the laboratory or the erosion of an unrelated inflammatory process (e.g., bacterial pneumonia) into a region of old, quiescent disease.

Atypical Mycobacteria

Mycobacteria other than TB frequently colonize the sputum of patients with chronic obstructive pulmonary disease, grow in gastric juice, or contaminate laboratory reagents, causing diagnostic confusion. On rare occasions these atypical organisms incite serious disease. As a group, atypicals differ from TB in several important ways: they are noncommunicable, do not involve pleural or extrapulmonary sites other than lymph nodes, and almost always produce indolent disease. Except for M. kansasii, they are poorly responsive to antibiotics. Diagnosis of atypical disease requires isolation of the same organism in moderate growth from multiple specimens of sputum.

Chest X-ray

It is often difficult to distinguish active from inactive disease by the routine chest film. Fluffy infiltrates and multiple small air-fluid levels indicate an acute process. Extensive calcification, fibrosis, or hilar retraction suggest inactivity. If clinical suspicion is strong, sputum should be examined, whatever the x-ray findings.

Tuberculosis most commonly involves apical and posterior segments of the upper lobes. It is rare for a tuberculous infiltrate to involve only the anterior segments of the upper lobes. (However, atypical mycobacteria and certain fungi can do this.) Lower lobe involvement can occur in any patient, due to endobronchial spread of infection from a ruptured cavity or an eroded peribronchial node.

Miliary tuberculosis can present with a negative chest x-ray, which only develops characteristic changes days to weeks later. If tuberculosis is strongly suspected, treatment should be initiated, despite an apparent lack of radiographic evidence.

DIAGNOSTIC WORKUP

Chest x-ray, including lordotic views if the apices are poorly visualized.

First AM sputum x 3 for direct and concentrated smears and cultures of AFB. Repeat using ultrasonic nebulizer to induce sputum if deep cough specimens of at least 5 ml are not obtained. Perform fiberoptic bronchoscopy with transbronchial biopsy to obtain tissue in difficult cases.

No further workup is necessary in the absence of clinical features suggesting extrapulmonary involvement. However, a search for extrapulmonary spread should be conducted in the presence of symptoms, physical findings, and abnormal routine laboratory data. Consider

> Spinal fluid analysis and culture, brain scan
> Urinalysis and culture, IVP
> Pleural fluid aspirate and pleural biopsy for stain and culture
> Tomography (conventional or computerized) of spinous and perispinous regions
> Biopsies and aspirates from peritoneal, pericardial, and joint spaces

Fluids produced by TB characteristically have high protein and low glucose concentrations. The predominant cell is usually, but not invariably, the small lymphocyte.

If clinical suspicion remains strong but definitive evidence is not at hand, treat first and await culture results.

MANAGEMENT

Principles of Antibiosis

Tuberculous organisms exist both in cavities, where numbers are large, division is rapid, and pH is modestly alkaline, and within closed caseous lesions and macrophages, where numbers are small, division is slow, and pH is modestly acidic. Cidal drugs used in therapy can be effective in an alkaline medium only (e.g., streptomycin, capreomycin), in an acidic medium only (e.g., pyrazinamide), or in both locations (e.g., isoniazid, rifampin). Other available drugs (ethambutol, ethionamide, cycloserine, and PAS) are inhibitory but not routinely cidal.

Effective chemotherapy is achieved when organisms in all environments receive the equivalent of one cidal drug. Populations of mycobacteria are not uniform in their susceptibility to antimycobacterial agents. Hence, isoniazid (INH) alone, rifampin alone, or the combination of pyrazinamide (PZA) and streptomycin alone would be sufficient therapy if drug resistance were not a problem. Unfortunately, resistance to one of the commonly used medications is spontaneously present in 1 in 10^4 to 1 in 10^7 organisms, depending upon the drug.

Since new infections and dormant closed foci contain as few as 10^2 to 10^4 organisms, INH alone is sufficient to sterilize them with little risk of inducing resistance; hence, it is effective in "prophylactic" regimens. Cavitary foci may contain 10^{10} mycobacteria, so that thousands of organisms may acquire resistance to any single drug; consequently, there is a substantial risk for the emergence of a resistant population.

Because effective antituberculous drugs operate through different mechanisms, the chance of an organism developing resistance to two drugs effective at that location is multiplicative and negligible.

First-line drugs for the treatment of tuberculosis are potent, easily administered, and have a low rate of adverse reactions. Second-line drugs are occasionally needed when dealing with organisms refractory to multiple first-line drugs. In general they are less effective, less convenient, and more frequently associated with toxic reactions.

Unlike the other antituberculous drugs, resistance to INH invitro does not necessarily imply lack of effectiveness in vivo. The explanation may be that INH is more effective at intracellular than at extracellular sites. Another possibility is that disease is usually caused by a mixed population of INH-sensitive and INH-resistant organisms, but only the INH-resistant organisms grow once INH has been started.

Initial Drug Regimens

Daily

In this country the large majority of patients developing tuberculosis have reactivated disease with organisms sensitive to all drugs. However, 20-60% of persons who contracted their disease in Africa, Asia, Central, or South America are infected with organisms resistant to one or more drugs. In the United States, the incidence of primary drug resistance exceeds 10% in urban centers where groups of such immigrants have congregated.

Although INH (300 mg, qd) plus ethambutol (15 mg/kg, qd) for 18-24 months is of established efficacy, the current treatment of choice for uncomplicated cases is INH (300 mg qd) and rifampin (600 mg qd), continued for a "short course" of 9-12 months.

Using this latter combination, a third drug is seldom required, since both drugs penetrate easily into all body spaces and are cidal everywhere. Nonetheless, it is rational to add either ethambutol or streptomycin for the first 6 weeks to 3 months if the patient is likely to have been infected with an organism resistant to INH, if cavities are massive, or if the patient is gravely ill, e.g., with miliary or CNS disease. (Seriously ill patients who cannot absorb oral medications present a problem; currently only INH and the "mycin" drugs can be given parenterally.) The development of recurrent disease after a full "short course" of INH and rifampin appears to be even less common than after treatment with other regimens given for longer periods.

Twice-Weekly Therapy

After an initial month to six weeks of daily therapy, twice-weekly therapy can be given successfully to most patients using INH and rifampin for an additional 8-11 months. Apart from convenience, such a schedule allows definitive monitoring of therapy in otherwise poorly compliant individuals. Other two-drug combinations, using either INH or rifampin together with ethambutol or streptomycin for 18 months, have also been successful.

"Ultrashort" (six-month) Course Regimens

Intensive therapy for even shorter periods than 9 months has recently been shown to be an effective alternative. An initial 2-month induction phase with four-drug therapy (rifampin, INH, PZA, and streptomycin) is integral to each of these. The continuation phase incorporates rifampin and INH for a four-month period. As a general rule these regimens should be applied only to relatively uncomplicated disease for extenuating social indications.

Table 35.1.

Drugs used in the treatment of mycobacterial disease, (daily adult dosage).

First Line		Second Line	
Isoniazid	5-10 mg/kg, up to 300 mg PO or IM	Capreomycin	12-15 mg/kg, up to 1 g IM
Ethambutol	15-25 mg/kg PO	Kanamycin	12-15 mg/kg, up to 1 g IM
Rifampin	10-15 mg/kg, up to 600 mg PO	Ethionamide	15 mg/kg, up to 1 g PO
Streptomycin	15 mg/kg, up to 1 g IM	PAS (aminosalicylic acid)	150 mg/kg, up to 12 g PO
Pyrazinamide	25 mg/kg, up to 2 g PO	Cycloserine	15 mg/kg, up to 1 g PO

Course of Treated Tuberculosis

Most febrile patients with adequately treated tuberculosis achieve a normal temperature after 3 weeks of therapy. Occasional patients with extensive cavitation spike sporadic fevers 12 weeks or more after therapy is initiated, but a trend toward normality is usually evident, and chest films show steady improvement. More prolonged fever suggests the development of drug resistance, drug allergy, or a superimposed bacterial process.

Very toxic patients may benefit from corticosteroid therapy (30 mg qd), as may those with tuberculous meningitis (decreases cerebral edema and adhesions) and pericarditis (possibly decreases the incidence of constrictive fibrosis). Sputum smears for acid-fast bacilli may be postive intermittently up to three months, but colony counts drop rapidly, and cultures are usually sterile after 8-12 weeks of continuous treatment. Recurrence is sufficiently rare after a properly completed course of antituberculous therapy that chest films taken later than six months after completion of treatment are not necessary.

Drug Resistance and Retreatment Regimens

If an appropriate combination of drugs is used continuously for an inadequate period of time, the organisms that emerge will usually remain sensitive to the initial regimen, and recrudescence will occur within the first several months after the drugs were stopped prematurely. However, if drugs are used erratically or in insufficient dosage, resistance to one or more of the drugs may occur. As a general rule, an organism will not develop resistance to a drug to which it has never been exposed.

Based on the principles of antibiosis previously outlined, one drug should never be added to a failing regimen; two new drugs are necessary, one cidal if possible. The regimen can be revised later, dropping unnecessary drugs as sensitivities return 2-3 months later. INH may be useful despite invitro resistance. In patients with suspected primary resistance, a regimen of INH, rifampin, and ethambutol is a particularly good choice, since resistance to either rifampin or ethambutol is rare.

Drug Toxicity and Interactions

The major risk of therapy with INH, rifampin, and PZA is hepatitis. The risk of combined therapy is only slightly higher than with each drug used individually.

Patients with preexisiting liver disease and older patients (especially females) appear to be at highest risk for INH hepatitis. Reactions are most likely in the first weeks of treatment but can occur at any time. Ten percent of persons will demonstrate a transient rise of hepatic transaminases (less than threefold) soon after starting INH, but only 5-10% of these will develop symptoms. Since little harm develops if INH is withdrawn promptly as symptoms arise, the patient should be educated as to the symptoms to watch for and followed without routine laboratory tests. (However, a baseline set of hepatic enzymes drawn before therapy may help determine the need for stopping the drug, should equivocal symptoms develop.) Similar recommendations seem warranted for patients on rifampin or PZA.

If a serious drug reaction is suspected (e.g., fever, hepatitis), all drugs should be discontinued for 4-7 days and reinstituted one-by-one, starting with the most suspicious of them. Otherwise, an extensive time on insufficient coverage can elapse before it is ascertained whether the symptoms are drug related at all, and if so, which drug is causative.

Special Problems

PZA routinely results in an elevation of uric acid (usually asymptomatic). INH slows the catabolism of diphenylhydantoin, sometimes requiring adjustment of dosage to avoid toxicity. Ethambutol in doses exceeding the standard dose of 15 mg/kg has cidal properties against TB but is also associated with optic neuritis. Rifampin accelerates metabolism of the coumarin drugs, oral contraceptives, corticosteroids, digitoxin, and oral hypoglycemics. In the presence of significant renal disease, the doses of ethambutol and streptomycin (but not INH or rifampin) need to be adjusted. All "mycin" antibiotics may cause 8th nerve damage - either auditory, vestibular, or both. In severe chronic hepatic disease, it seems unwise to use both INH and rifampin in the same regimen.

Surgery

Drug therapy is both necessary and sufficient in the vast majority of cases. However, surgical intervention (including excision of infected tissues, closure of bronchopleural fistulae, or obliteration of infected pleural spaces) should be considered in the following circumstances: 1) advancing localized disease unresponsive to chemotherapy or resistant to feasible regimens, 2) complications of tuberculous infection, including life-threatening hemoptysis and bronchopleural fistula, 3) localized infection with atypical mycobacteria, unresponsive to antibiotics, and 4) disabling symptoms due to localized damage by previous TB (e.g., bronchiectasis).

To control endobronchitis and minimize the risk of dehiscence and fistula formation, surgery in patients with active disease must be performed under coverage of at least two weeks of an effective antibiotic regimen, whenever possible.

Tuberculous empyema generally responds well to drug therapy alone. Intercostal drainage by tube thoracostomy is discouraged because of the risk of bacterial contamination. (This attitude may be an inappropriate residual of the preantibiotic era.) Tuberculous bronchopleural fistula, however, should be treated both with TB chemotherapy and intercostal catheter drainage, adding antibacterial agents as necessary.

Need for Isolation

Untreated, smear-positive, coughing patients are the most likely to aerosolize infective particles. Smear-negative patients are little, if any, more infective than patients with sterile cultures and need not be isolated once chemotherapy is begun. However, patients who continue to cough should do so into disposable tissues. Hospitalized smear-positive patients spread disease by talking, coughing, and sneezing and should be confined initially to a room having adequate ventilation, with air flowing unidirectionally from the room to the outdoors. An ultraviolet light directed toward the ceiling helps to sterilize the air. Masks should be worn by the patient or by the staff during this isolation period.

Once placed on effective chemotherapy, infectivity declines precipitously because 1) the number of organisms diminishes, 2) the frequency of coughing decreases, and 3) aerosolized organisms may be rendered non-viable by drugs highly concentrated as water evaporates from the droplet nucleus.

No definitive information as to exact criteria for discontinuance of isolation is available. However, when cough decreases, when the patient improves subjectively, and when the number of organisms in serial sputum smears declines, the risk appears acceptably low, despite the continued presence of organisms in the sputum. Isolation should probably continue if these criteria are violated, even after a lengthy period on therapy. However, based on epidemiologic evidence of PPD-negative household contacts re-exposed to smear-positive patients, noninfectiousness has usually been conferred by two weeks of drug treatment. Restriction of activity, special diets, etc. are of no value and should be discouraged.

Prophylaxis

Isonazid (INH)

According to criteria of the American Thoracic Society, the following should receive (therapeutic) "prophylaxis" with one year of INH (300 mg qd), in descending order of highest risk: 1) Household contacts and close associates of a recently diagnosed case of active TB, 2) Positive skin test reactors with chest x-rays suggestive of nonprogressive tuberculous disease who are bacteriologically negative and who have not previously received chemotherapy, 3) Newly infected persons, defined as patients who have "converted" their skin test reaction from positive to negative within the past two years (see definition of conversion, p. 270), 4) Positive skin test reaction plus one or more of the following risk factors:

a. prolonged therapy with corticosteroids or immunosuppressive therapy
b. some hematologic or reticuloendothelial malignancies (e.g., leukemia, Hodgkin's disease)
c. unstable diabetes mellitus
d. silicosis
e. gastrectomy

5) <u>Persons under the age of 35 with positive skin test</u>

The last recommendation is the most controversial. Few experts disagree that children and adolescents should receive prophylaxis, since the liklihood of recent infection is higher, defenses are lower, and the risk of INH hepatitis is minimal. With advancing age, it becomes less certain whether the risk of activating tuberculosis outweighs the inconvenience and potential toxicity of the regimen.

Alternative Drug Regimens for Prophylaxis

In persons exposed to an active case of INH-resistant disease, there are several options:

1) Do nothing and observe (not recommended).
2) Prescribe INH in the hope that in vivo sensitivity is preserved, despite in vitro test results.
3) Substitute rifampin.

There is no proven alternative to INH in patients already infected with TB. However, many physicians prescribe rifampin (600 mg) for one year in its place, based on the knowledge that both are cidal drugs and that development of rifampin-resistant organisms is unlikely, due to the small numbers involved. Nonetheless, important questions regarding toxicity, optimal duration, and emergence of resistance remain.

BCG Vaccination

Even if efficacious, BCG is potentially useful only in noninfected (PPD-negative) persons. BCG is rarely used in this country since 1) the large majority of active cases of TB occur in patients already infected at some time in the distant past, 2) the risk of exposure is relatively low, and 3) identified patients with active disease who received drug therapy are noncontagious.

Reporting

All active or strongly suspected cases of tuberculosis must be reported promptly to the local health department. In many instances, these workers can then identify and treat contacts of the index case, as well as provide the follow-up needed for cure.

FUNGAL DISEASES OF THE LUNG

Five categories account for the majority of pulmonary fungal disease: histoplasmosis, blastomycosis, coccidioidomycosis, cryptococcosis, and aspergillosis. No attempt to exhaustively cover this complex object can be presented here. However, a few features germane to the hospitalized patient are worth emphasizing.

Histoplasmosis

In North America acute histoplasmosis is seen almost exclusively in its endemic area, the east-central United States. Its manifestations depend on the intensity of exposure and the ability of the subject to cope with infection. If exposure is light, symptoms are few. In its most common presentation, mild flu-like symptoms arise approximately two weeks after exposure and abate without treatment. Patchy pneumonitis and hilar adenopathy are characteristic. Residual disease often takes the form of multiple parenchymal granulomata and hilar node calcification. Larger exposures may cause a more impressive, but again usually self-limited, syndrome. Fever and diffuse x-ray changes dominate the clinical picture.

Cavitating histoplasmosis resembles tuberculosis in its radiographic appearance, its predilection for the upper lobes, and its indolent clinical course. It arises not from reactivation, however, but from a primary infection of previously diseased lung. Antifungal chemotherapy may be required. Disseminated disease in adults is most common among elderly men and immunosuppressed patients. Symptomatic involvement of extrapulmonary tissues such as skin, mucous membranes, and hepatic and hematopoetic tissues account for the marked constitutional symptoms that characterize this disease. The definitive diagnosis of histoplasmosis rests on the demonstration of the fungus in affected tissue, where it appears as tightly crowded yeast forms within an engulfing macrophage. Serologic studies can require weeks for completion. Skin tests are of no value. Histoplasmosis responds both to oral ketoconazole and to intravenous amphotericin. The latter agent is most appropriate for hospitalized patients.

Blastomycosis

Endemic to the southern United States, blastomycosis is also prevalent in the northern midwest. It is more frequent in rural than urban areas. Acute blastomycosis can present as an acute pneumonia with high fever, basilar infiltrates, and flu-like symptomatology. More commonly, however, it has an indolent presentation, similar to tuberculosis. Involvement of skin, bone, prostate, and central nervous system are unusual but do occur. Unlike histoplasmosis, the diagnosis of blastomycosis can often be established by the examination of sputum or other involved tissue after 10% KOH digestion or cytologic study (Papanicolaou's technique). Treatment of blastomycosis is determined by the severity of illness. Many cases resolve spontaneously without intervention. Oral ketoconazole is acceptable if the disease is relatively mild and does not involve the central nervous system. In the latter instance, intravenous amphotericin is more appropriate.

Coccidioidomycosis

Coccidioidomycosis affects patients from a restricted geographic range that includes central California and the desert Southwest. In endemic regions exposure is almost universal, but most exposures do not come to clinical notice. A small percentage of persons will develop a flu-like illness characterized by fever, chills, cough, dyspnea, arthralgia, and skin rash. Chest infiltrates are very common, even without associated symptomatology. Hilar adenopathy and pleural effusions may be part of the radiographic picture. The great majority of patients recover uneventfully from primary "coccy," but a few go on to persistent or disseminated variants. Identified high-risk populations are darkly pigmented, particularly Blacks and Filipinos. The height of the complement fixation (CF) and immunodiffusion titers correlate with the severity of the disease and the risk of dissemination.

Failure of the acute syndrome to resolve over several weeks may signal the presence of refractory, progressive disease and the need for antibiotic therapy. Pulmonary findings include progressive destructive pneumonitis and unifocal or multifocal nodular disease. Pulmonary coccidioidomas are often peripherally located and thin walled. Although they seldom are associated with symptoms, pleurisy and even empyema may result. The development of symptoms, progressive infiltration, or high and rising CF titers portend a difficult course and mandate treatment. Amphotercin is generally selected for serious cases, whereas ketoconazole may suffice for minimally symptomatic disease.

Disseminated coccy, generally a disease of those with defective cell-mediated immunity, is characterized by disease in the skin, joints, bone, or meningeal space. It is a life-threatening disorder that always demands aggressive treatment. Meningeal disease appears to require intracisternal amphotericin for effective control.

Cryptococcosis

Cryptococcosis has no geographical predilection. In human tissues it proliferates as a yeast with a thick capsule that aids in its identification. The cryptococcus gains entry via pulmonary tissues and often remains confined to the lung. The inflammatory reaction it evokes can be indolent and is usually histiocytic (granulomatous) in nature. Radiographic evidence for pulmonary involvement is protean, presenting either as single or multiple peripheral nodules, a mass (toruloma), or an infiltrate. Miliary dissemination of cryptococcus throughout the lung occurs rarely but can produce a devastating syndrome.

Persons with diseases of depressed cell-mediated immunity are not only more likely to manifest disease but also are at greatest risk for dissemination to the meninges, kidney, and other less common extrapulmonary sites. A small fraction of patients with cryptococcal meningitis have no obvious T-lymphocyte disorder but can be shown to have a selectively weakened response to cryptococcal antigens.

Identification of the cryptococcus in involved tissues is not difficult when the appropriate special stains are used but is not easily demonstrated in tissues or in body fluids by usual techniques. PAS or mucicarmine stains should be ordered specially if crypto is suspected. Serologic studies can be of great assistance. Crypto polysaccharide antigen can be used to detect the organism in the spinal fluid, urine, and serum. Counter immunoelectrophoresis is more reliable than latex agglutination for this purpose. High titers in the cerebrospinal fluid are a poor prognostic sign.

Without question, disseminated cryptococcosis, cryptococcal meningitis, and symptomatic pulmonary disease should be treated. The combination of amphotericin and flucytosine is the therapy of choice. There is no convincing evidence that asymptomatic pulmonary nodules need to be treated in the absence of dissemination or predisposition thereto.

Aspergillosis

Like cryptococcus, aspergillus has no geographic predilection but, unlike crypto, takes the form of a mycelium with side arms that branch at an acute 45° angle. It is perhaps the most commonly encountered fungus in hospitalized patients, generating problems of three quite different kinds.

Allergic bronchopulmonary aspergillosis is a varied syndrome that may involve episodic fever, cough, bronchospasm, evanescent pulmonary infiltrates, and constitutional complaints. Mucoid impaction of the central bronchi, identified by the radiographic appearance of a "cluster of grapes" or "gloved finger," is caused by inspissation of the unusually thick mucus evoked by this fungal saprophyte. The disease can be identified by staining aspergilli in mucous plugs, but laboratory studies are more reliable. Eosinophilia and high levels of IgE are usually present in the serum. Delayed skin hypersensitivity to aspergillus is so characteristic that its absence should call the diagnosis into question. Serum precipitins to aspergillus are also present in the great majority of cases. Response is excellent to corticosteroids and bronchodilator therapy.

Aspergillomas (fungus balls) are agglomerations of mycelial elements, mucus, and cellular debris that colonize the preexisting cavities of healed tuberculosis or emphysema. Usually asymptomatic, they generally cause trouble by mimicking a neoplasm or by causing hemoptysis. Constitutional complaints are unusual. Radiographically, thickened cavity walls and mobility of the mycetoma on repositioning are characteristic. The typical radiographic appearance together with serum precipitins (usually very high titer) establish the diagnosis. Treatment depends on manifestations. Recurrent hemoptysis, especially if massive, may require resection. Corticosteroids are rarely helpful.

Invasive aspergillosis is a devastating disease of the immune-compromised host. Although patients with impaired granulocyte count and function are the most highly susceptible, this almost universally fatal disease can occur in any patient with marked compromise of immune function. Renal transplant recipients are distressingly frequent victims. Although often widespread, invasive aspergillosis almost invariably manifests prominently in the lung. One hallmark of this disease in the lung is blood vessel invasion, infarction, and patchy necrosis of lung parenchyma. Hemoptysis, peripheral cavitation, and chest pain are therefore unusually common, in addition to the other features of pneumonitis. The diagnosis of invasive aspergillosis must usually await the availability of lung tissue to establish the diagnosis. Ancillary tests are not helpful. Although the pace of this disease is highly variable, a fatal outcome is virtually always the endpoint in patients who do not recover lost host defenses over the period of treatment. Nonetheless recent experience has shown that a few fortunate patients will survive if therapy with amphotercin is begun early enough, in conjunction with effective treatment of the primary disorder.

Nocardia and Actinomycosis

These unusual infections share several clinical and microbiological features and are therefore often considered together as "higher bacteria." Neither fits comfortably into a classification of either bacterial or fungal disease. Both tend to produce indolent infections and demonstrate morphologic characteristics of fungi (mycelial formation), but both respond (albeit slowly) to appropriate antibacterial chemotherapy.

Nocardia can infect any host, but most often affects middle-aged and elderly males, particularly those with abnormal lungs, patients with T-cell immune defects, and patients with alveolar proteinosis. The inflammatory reaction tends to be a localized suppurative process, complicated by dense fibrosis or abscess formation. Airway distortion, airway compression, atelectasis, and sinus tract formation are not rare. Pleural effusions are not a recognized part of the disease spectrum. Acute as well as chronic presentations are common. Metastatic infections are most likely to seed the brain, skin, or subcutaneous tissues.

Nocardia, unlike actinomycosis, can often be recovered from sputum samples, where its fine branching filaments stain Gram positive when they remain intact. Although the organism may be weakly acid-fast, this is highly variable. Tissue specimens must be stained with Gram and Giemsa techniques to demonstrate the organism, as routine H and E preparations are not effective. Nocardia is generally less responsive to antibiotics than is actinomycosis, requiring prolonged high-dose sulfonamide treatment for response. A substantial fraction of patients fail treatment. Trimethoprim-sulfamethoxazole is the current drug of choice, with minocycline as a second-line alternative in sulfa-allergic patients.

Actinomycosis differs from Nocardia in a number of important respects. It shows no predilection for the disadvantaged host. Rather, it tends to develop after aspiration from the oropharynx of a patient with periodontal or tonsillar disease. Although actinomycosis of the lung can present as a diffuse and acute alveolitis, it more often is a localized process, complicated by cavitation, chest wall inflammation, pleural effusion, empyema, and sinus tract formation. Unlike Nocardia, localized extension across anatomic boundaries to adjacent tissues is common, whereas metastatic involvement of other vital organs is highly unusual.

The diagnosis of actinomycosis may be difficult without tissue biopsy and careful culturing technique. Macroscopic "sulfur granules" in expectorated sputum (mycelial agglomerations) strongly suggest the diagnosis, but anaerobic culture is required to define their etiology. Like Nocardia, actinomycetes tend to form filaments that stain Gram positive. However an acid-fast stain may distinguish these organims, since actinomycetes are unlikely to be acid-fast if adequately decolorized. In tissue, actinomycetes tend to stain well with H and E, again a departure from Nocardia. Actinomycosis also responds differently to antibiotics, being quite sensitive to a number of drugs. Although penicillin remains the treatment of choice, most antibiotics effective against anaerobic infection tend to be effective. Tetracycline, clindamycin, and chloramphenicol are perhaps the best alternatives for the penicillin-allergic patient. Therapy should be continued for at least 3 months and preferably for 12-18 months. Treatment failures are less common than in nocardiosis.

SUGGESTED READINGS

Tuberculosis

1. American College of Chest Physicians National Consensus Conference on Tuberculosis. Chest 1985;87(2):115S-149S (Suppl).

2. Dutt AK, Stead WW. Present chemotherapy for tuberculosis. J. Infect. Dis. 1982;146:698-704.

3. Glassroth J, Robins AG, Snider DE. Tuberculosis in the 1980's. N. Engl. J. Med. 1980;302:1441-50.

4. Johnston RF, Wildrick KH. The impact of chemotherapy on the care of patients with tuberculosis. Am. Rev. Respir. Dis. 1974;109:636-64.

5. Snider DE Jr, et al. Standard therapy for tuberculosis, 1985. Chest 1985;87:117S-24S.

Fungal Disease

1. Cohen J. Anti fungal chemotherapy. Lancet 1982;2:532-37.

2. Kerkering TM, Duma RJ, Shadomy S. The evolution of pulmonary cryptococcosis: Clinical implications from a study of 41 patients with and without compromising host factors. Ann. Intern. Med. 1981;94:611-16.

3. Palmer DL, Harvey RL, Wheeler JK. Diagnostic and therapeutic considerations in nocardia asteroides infection. Medicine 1974;53:391-401.

4. Pennington JE. Aspergillus lung disease. Med. Clin. North Am. 1980;64:475-90.

5. Stamm AM, Dismukes WE. Current therapy of pulmonary and disseminated fungal diseases. Chest 1983;83:911-17.

Index